HEALTH CARE ISSUES, COSTS AND ACCESS

MEDIGAP

A PRIMER ON MEDICARE SUPPLEMENT INSURANCE

HEALTH CARE ISSUES, COSTS AND ACCESS

Additional books in this series can be found on Nova's website under the Series tab.

Additional E-books in this series can be found on Nova's website under the E-book tab.

HEALTH CARE ISSUES, COSTS AND ACCESS

MEDIGAP

A PRIMER ON MEDICARE SUPPLEMENT INSURANCE

JOHNY P. HUGHES
EDITOR

New York

For permission to use material from this book please contact us:
Telephone 631-231-7269; Fax 631-231-8175
Web Site: http://www.novapublishers.com

Additional color graphics may be available in the e-book version of this book.

Library of Congress Cataloging-in-Publication Data

ISBN: 978-1-62417-279-3

Published by Nova Science Publishers, Inc. † New York

Contents

Preface

Medicare is a nationwide health insurance program for individuals aged 65 and over and certain disabled individuals. The basic Medicare benefit package provides broad protection against the costs of many, primarily acute, health care services. However, Medicare beneficiaries may still have significant additional costs, including copayments, coinsurance, deductibles, and the full cost of services that are not covered by Medicare. In 2008, about 17% of Medicare beneficiaries purchased the private supplemental insurance known as Medigap to fill some of the cost gaps left by Original Medicare. This book provides an overview of Medigap insurance with a focus on the history of Medigap legislation; the various types of Medigap plans; consumer protections awarded to Medigap beneficiaries; and the requirements facing the insurance providers and the National Association of Insurance Carriers (NAIC).

Chapter 1 – Medicare is a nationwide health insurance program for individuals aged 65 and over and certain disabled individuals. The basic Medicare benefit package (termed "Original Medicare" in this report) provides broad protection against the costs of many, primarily acute, health care services. However, Medicare beneficiaries may still have significant additional costs, including copayments, coinsurance, deductibles, and the full cost of services that are not covered by Medicare. In 2008, about 17% of Medicare beneficiaries purchased the private supplemental insurance known as Medigap to fill some of the cost gaps left by Original Medicare.

All Medigap plans cover some percentage of Medicare's cost-sharing. Some plans offer additions to these basics, including various combinations of greater coverage of Medicare cost-sharing, and care associated with foreign travel emergencies. The most popular plans are the most comprehensive, and cover all deductibles, copayments, and coinsurance not covered by Medicare. Medigap generally does not cover medical treatments not covered by Medicare, although it does extend coverage for certain covered services, such as coverage for additional hospital days beyond the Medicare benefit limit. Medigap is financed through beneficiary payments to the private insurance firms.

Federal law requires that Medigap insurers observe many consumer protections. Consumer protections are especially strong during open enrollment, which is a six-month period that begins for most individuals during the month they turn 65. During this period, individuals are protected against

- insurers refusing to sell them any Medigap policy that the insurer offers,
- insurers setting premiums based on the individual's health, and
- insurers imposing waiting times on the start of the policy, other than a maximum of a six-month waiting period for preexisting conditions.

Following the open-enrollment period, beneficiaries have other rights in limited situations, such as when they move to a different state. Guaranteed issue (or the right to buy a plan, to have the plan's premium not depend on health status, and in some cases to have the plan start coverage of preexisting conditions immediately) is one such right. The right of guaranteed renewability is available in a wide variety of situations, and genetic discrimination is forbidden. Moreover, Medigap insurers must pay out at least 65% (and sometimes 75%) of total premiums as claims to the beneficiaries. Recent data show that Medigap premiums vary by states and other factors. A relatively small number of insurance firms sell Medigap plans. In addition, Medigap beneficiaries are concentrated in certain areas of the country and are more likely to have lower incomes than those holding employer-sponsored retiree health insurance. The Patient Protection and Affordable Care Act (P.L. 111-148 as amended by P.L. 111-152, ACA) requests that the Secretary of Health and Human Services ask the National Association of Insurance Commissioners to review and revise existing standards to examine greater cost-sharing for Medigap beneficiaries. In addition, the President's 2013 budget proposal would provide incentives to increase cost-sharing. One rationale for these proposals is that beneficiaries on average reduce their use of medical care following an increase in cost-sharing. This decrease in medical care by Medicare beneficiaries could reduce Medicare expenditures and the federal deficit. On the other hand, if these reductions in medical care ultimately lower health status, the individuals might require more treatments or more expensive care. This report provides a broad overview of Medigap insurance. The report covers the history of Medigap legislation, the various types of Medigap plans, consumer protections awarded to Medigap beneficiaries, and the requirements facing the insurance providers and the NAIC. Following an empirical description of Medigap markets, the report discusses proposals related to the percentages of a Medigap insurer's revenue that is returned as benefits to the policy holders and Medigap cost-sharing requirements.

Chapter 2 – This offcial government guide has important information about the following:

- What is a Medigap (Medicare Supplement Insurance) policy
- What Medigap policies cover
- Your rights to buy a Medigap policy
- How to buy a Medigap policy

This guide can help if you're thinking about buying a Medigap policy or already have one.

Chapter 3 – Medicare is a federal insurance program that pays for covered health care services of qualified beneficiaries. It was established in 1965 under Title XVIII of the Social Security Act as a federal entitlement program to provide health insurance to individuals 65 and older, and has been expanded over the years to include permanently disabled individuals under 65. Medicare, which consists of four parts (A-D), covers hospitalizations, physician services, prescription drugs, skilled nursing facility care, home health visits, and hospice care, among other services.

Generally, individuals are eligible for Medicare if they or their spouse worked for at least 40 quarters in Medicare-covered employment, are 65 years old, and are a citizen or permanent resident of the United States. Individuals may also qualify for coverage if they are a younger person with a permanent disability, have End-Stage Renal disease (permanent kidney failure requiring dialysis or transplant), or have amyotrophic lateral sclerosis (ALS, Lou Gehrig's disease). In addition, individuals with one or more specified lung diseases or types of cancer who lived for six months during a specified period prior to diagnosis in an area subject to a public health emergency declaration by the Environmental Protection Agency (EPA) as of June 17, 2009, are also deemed entitled to benefits under Part A and eligible to enroll in Part B.

In FY2012, the program will cover approximately 50 million persons (41 million aged and 9 million disabled) at a total cost of about $576 billion, accounting for approximately 3.7% of GDP. Medicare is an entitlement program, which means that it is required to pay for covered services provided to eligible persons so long as specific criteria are met.

Since 1965, the Medicare program has undergone considerable change. During the 111th Congress, the Patient Protection and Affordable Care Act (ACA; P.L. 111-148) and the Health Care and Education Affordability Reconciliation Act of 2010 (the Reconciliation Act, or HCERA; P.L. 111-152) were signed into law. They made numerous changes to the Medicare program that modify provider reimbursements, provide incentives to increase the quality and efficiency of care, and enhance certain Medicare benefits.

However, in the absence of congressional action, the Medicare program will be unsustainable in the long run. The Hospital Insurance (Part A) trust fund has been estimated to become insolvent in 2024. And although the Supplementary Medical Insurance (Parts B and D) trust fund is financed in large part through federal general revenues and cannot become insolvent, Medicare spending growth will put increasing strains on Congress's competing priorities.

The 112th Congress may continue to debate the recent changes to Medicare and may also consider additional legislative action ranging from technical corrections to broader structural changes. Additionally, Congress may consider legislative action to address the 2013-2021 automatic Medicare spending reductions under the Budget Control Act of 2011 (BCA; P.L. 112-25).

In: Medigap
Editor: Johny P. Hughes

ISBN: 978-1-62417-279-3

Chapter 1

Medigap: A Primer*

Carol Rapaport

Summary

Medicare is a nationwide health insurance program for individuals aged 65 and over and certain disabled individuals. The basic Medicare benefit package (termed "Original Medicare" in this report) provides broad protection against the costs of many, primarily acute, health care services. However, Medicare beneficiaries may still have significant additional costs, including copayments, coinsurance, deductibles, and the full cost of services that are not covered by Medicare. In 2008, about 17% of Medicare beneficiaries purchased the private supplemental insurance known as Medigap to fill some of the cost gaps left by Original Medicare.

All Medigap plans cover some percentage of Medicare's cost-sharing. Some plans offer additions to these basics, including various combinations of greater coverage of Medicare cost-sharing, and care associated with foreign travel emergencies. The most popular plans are the most comprehensive, and cover all deductibles, copayments, and coinsurance not covered by Medicare. Medigap generally does not cover medical treatments not covered by Medicare, although it does extend coverage for certain covered services, such as coverage for additional hospital days beyond the Medicare benefit limit. Medigap is financed through beneficiary payments to the private insurance firms.

* This is an edited, reformatted and augmented version of Congressional Research Service, Publication No. R42745, dated September 19, 2012.

Federal law requires that Medigap insurers observe many consumer protections. Consumer protections are especially strong during open enrollment, which is a six-month period that begins for most individuals during the month they turn 65. During this period, individuals are protected against

- insurers refusing to sell them any Medigap policy that the insurer offers,
- insurers setting premiums based on the individual's health, and
- insurers imposing waiting times on the start of the policy, other than a maximum of a six-month waiting period for preexisting conditions.

Following the open-enrollment period, beneficiaries have other rights in limited situations, such as when they move to a different state. Guaranteed issue (or the right to buy a plan, to have the plan's premium not depend on health status, and in some cases to have the plan start coverage of preexisting conditions immediately) is one such right. The right of guaranteed renewability is available in a wide variety of situations, and genetic discrimination is forbidden. Moreover, Medigap insurers must pay out at least 65% (and sometimes 75%) of total premiums as claims to the beneficiaries. Recent data show that Medigap premiums vary by states and other factors. A relatively small number of insurance firms sell Medigap plans. In addition, Medigap beneficiaries are concentrated in certain areas of the country and are more likely to have lower incomes than those holding employer-sponsored retiree health insurance. The Patient Protection and Affordable Care Act (P.L. 111-148 as amended by P.L. 111-152, ACA) requests that the Secretary of Health and Human Services ask the National Association of Insurance Commissioners to review and revise existing standards to examine greater cost-sharing for Medigap beneficiaries. In addition, the President's 2013 budget proposal would provide incentives to increase cost-sharing. One rationale for these proposals is that beneficiaries on average reduce their use of medical care following an increase in cost-sharing. This decrease in medical care by Medicare beneficiaries could reduce Medicare expenditures and the federal deficit. On the other hand, if these reductions in medical care ultimately lower health status, the individuals might require more treatments or more expensive care. This report provides a broad overview of Medigap insurance. The report covers the history of Medigap legislation, the various types of Medigap plans, consumer protections awarded to Medigap beneficiaries, and the requirements facing the insurance providers and the NAIC. Following an empirical description of Medigap markets, the report discusses proposals related to the percentages of a Medigap insurer's revenue that is returned as benefits to the policy holders and Medigap cost-sharing requirements.

Introduction

Medicare is a nationwide health insurance program for individuals aged 65 and over and certain disabled individuals. The basic Medicare benefit package (termed "Original Medicare" in this report) provides broad protection against the costs of many, primarily acute, health care services. However, Medicare beneficiaries may still have significant additional costs. Medicare requires beneficiaries to pay part of the cost for most covered services, provides only limited protection for some services (e.g., medical costs incurred outside of the United States), and provides no protection for other services (e.g., custodial long-term care, hearing aids, and dentures). Furthermore, unlike most large group health insurance policies, Original Medicare contains no upper ("catastrophic") limit on out-of-pocket expenses. As a result, Medicare beneficiaries have the potential to incur high out-of-pocket costs for their health care. Most Medicare beneficiaries therefore have some form of (private or public) additional coverage to supplement some or all of their out-of-pocket costs for Medicare benefits. *Medigap* is one form of private supplemental coverage; Medigap fills some of the cost gaps left by Medicare, such as deductibles, coinsurance, and copayments. [1] In order to be eligible to purchase Medigap, individuals must be

- enrolled in both Part A (Hospital Insurance) and Part B (Supplementary Medical Insurance) of Original Medicare, and
- not enrolled in Medicare Advantage (an HMO-type plan).

Medigap is financed through beneficiary payments to private insurance firms, although retirees may have premiums paid on their behalf by their former employers. There are no government contributions toward Medigap premiums. This report provides an overview of Medigap. After a review of Medicare coverage, the report covers the ways in which Medicare is supplemented. A discussion of the Medigap plans includes standardized plans, prestandardized plans, older standardized plans available for renewal only, plans in states with Medigap waivers, SELECT plans, and high-deductible plans. The analysis then covers various consumer protections, and the requirements for the insurance companies that offer Medigap. Next, the role of the National Association of Insurance Commissioners (NAIC), a nongovernmental advisory body, is discussed. The report then provides an empirical picture of Medigap markets. The report concludes with a discussion of two current policy issues. First, how much of the total collected premiums might each insurer be expected to return to its beneficiaries as payment for claims? Second, what is the potential effect on Medicare spending and the federal deficit of increasing the share of health care costs that the individual must pay out of his or her own pocket? Individuals on average reduce their use of medical care following an increase in the price of care. The decrease in medical care by Medicare beneficiaries could lead to a reduction in aggregate Medicare expenditures and a reduction in the deficit. On the other hand, the beneficiaries could experience deteriorations in health status if they reduce their use of medical services, which could lead to an ultimate increase in the amount and cost of necessary care, and an increase in Medicare spending and the deficit.

Medicare Coverage

Medicare consists of four parts:

- Part A, Hospital Insurance (HI), covers inpatient hospital services, skilled nursing care, some home health care, and hospice care.
- Part B, Supplementary Medical Insurance (SMI), covers physician and non-physician practitioner services, outpatient services, some home health, durable medical equipment, clinical laboratory and other diagnostic tests, preventive services, Part B drugs and biologics, and other medical services.
- Part C, Medicare Advantage (MA, a private plan option for beneficiaries), covers all Part A and Part B services, except hospice care.[2]
- Part D covers prescription drug benefit.

Together, Part A and Part B of Medicare comprise Original Medicare, which covers benefits on a fee-for-service (FFS) basis. Currently, most Medicare beneficiaries choose Original Medicare, obtaining covered services through the providers of their choice with Medicare paying its share of the bill for each rendered service. Alternatively, about one-fourth of all beneficiaries choose to enroll in a Medicare Advantage plan. Most individuals aged 65 and over are automatically eligible for premium-free Part A based on either their own or their spouses' work history.[3] Enrollment in Part B is voluntary and requires a premium. Everyone enrolled in Part A and/or Part B can elect Part D, with premiums varying by the Part D plans. **Table 1** provides a brief overview of the coverage offered under Medicare Part A and Part B, along with the associated cost-sharing.[4]

Table 1. Select Original Medicare Cost-Sharing Levels, 2012

Benefits	Cost-Sharing for Beneficiaries
Medicare Part A	
Inpatient hospital stay, per benefit period	
Days 1-60	$1,156 deductible
Days 61-90	$289 per day
Lifetime reserve days (up to 60)	$578 per day
Additional days	100%
Hospice care	
Care	$0
Prescriptions	Up to $5
Inpatient respite care	5%
Skilled nursing facility care, per benefit period	
Days 1-20	$0
Days 21-100	$144.50 per day
After day 100	100%
Part A deductible	(see hospital, Days 1-60, above)
Medicare Part B	
Medical and other services (includes physicians)	20%
Outpatient treatment of mental health services	40%
Excess charges	No coverage of excess charges
Part B deductible	$140
Blood	100% of the cost of reimbursement for the actual expense of blood (if any) and for the processing and service charges for the first 3 pints inside and/or outside the hospital; copayment after the first three pints outside the hospital
Foreign travel emergency	No coverage of foreign travel emergencies
Out-of-pocket limit	No out of pocked limit

Sources: Centers for Medicare & Medicaid Services, *Medicare and You*, 2012, pp. 31-54 and pp. 59-65, http://www.medicare.gov/publications/pubs/pdf/10050.pdf, and Centers for Medicare & Medicaid Services, *FAQ: Frequently Asked Questions About Medicare*, October 27, 2011, https://questions.medicare.gov/ app/answers/ detail/ a_id/2309/kw/ 2012%20DEDUCTABLE.

Notes: Cost-sharing is waived for certain screenings and preventive services. The deductible is waived for home health services, community health services, preventive services, and some other services. A benefit period begins the day the beneficiary is admitted to a hospital or skilled nursing facility, and ends when the beneficiary has not received hospital or skilled nursing care for 60 consecutive days. Excess charges are the difference between the Medicare approved amount and actual charges, subject to charge limitations set by Medicare or state law. There is a 190-day limit on lifetime inpatient mental health care days.

Medicare does not cover all medical goods and services, including custodial long-term care, routine dental care, dentures, vision care, cosmetic surgery, acupuncture, most care received in other countries, charges above what Medicare reimburses, and hearing aids, among others.[5] There is no out-of-pocket limit under Original Medicare. Alternatively, some beneficiaries are enrolled in Medicare Advantage (MA), which is also known as Part C. These beneficiaries obtain all covered Medicare services except hospice care through private policies, such as health maintenance organizations (HMOs). Some Part C enrollees may be offered additional benefits beyond what is available in Original Medicare; the scope of additional benefits varies by the health insurance plan. MA plans may include drugs through MA-PD (prescription drug) plans. Individuals who are enrolled in an MA plan may not be sold a Medigap plan.[6]

Supplementing Medicare

Many individuals have additional health insurance coverage to help pay for some of the costs that Medicare does not cover. **Figure 1** presents the breakdown across supplemental coverage types in 2008.[7]

Only 10% of the Medicare population had no supplemental coverage; these individuals relied solely on Original Medicare. The largest group of individuals (33%) of all Medicare beneficiaries received supplemental coverage from their employers. The next largest group of individuals (24%) were enrolled in Medicare Advantage. Medigap (17%) and Medicaid (15%) were other sources of supplemental insurance.[8]

Medigap Plans

Medigap policies are sold in both the individual and the group health insurance markets. Whether purchased in the individual or the group market, each Medigap policy covers one individual.[9]

Plans are identified by letter, and each plan is associated with a specific benefit package. For example, all Plan As have the same benefit package. The term "plan" refers to all the Medigap insurance contracts with a common benefit package, and the term "policy" refers to an insurance contract sold by an insurer to a beneficiary (e.g., United Healthcare's Plan A).

Federal law governing the sale of Medigap plans is contained in section 1882 of the Social Security Act. This section of the report first provides a history of Medigap legislation and then characterizes the various Medigap plans.

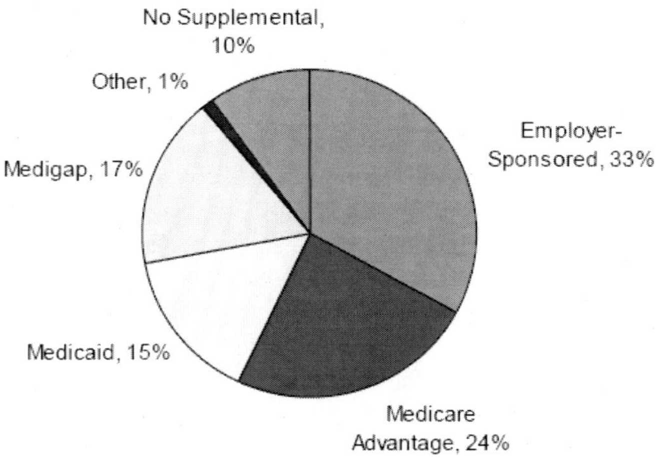

Source: Juliette Cubanski, Jennifer Huang, and Anthony Damico, et al., *Medicare Chartbook*, The Henry J. Kaiser Family Foundation, November 2010, p. 60, http://www.kff.org/medicare/upload/8103.pdf.

Notes: Data are from the Medicare Current Beneficiary Survey, Access to Care File, 2008. Employer-sponsored insurance includes retiree drug subsidies and TRICARE (the military health care program). All of the pie pieces are mutually exclusive in that once an individual has one type of supplemental insurance (or none), he or she cannot have another type. Supplemental coverage was assigned in the following order: (1) Medicare Advantage, (2) Medicaid, (3) Employer-Sponsored Insurance, (4) Medigap, (5) Other, and (6) No supplemental coverage. Individuals with more than one source of coverage were assigned to the category that appears highest in the ordering.

Figure 1. Sources of Supplemental Coverage Among Medicare Beneficiaries, 2008.

History of Medigap Statutes

Health insurance regulation largely has been and continues to be the province of the states; Medigap is a partial exception.[10] Medigap reform began in 1980, and changes over the years can be characterized along several dimensions. What began as voluntary standards governing the behavior of insurers increasingly became requirements. Consumer protections were continuously strengthened, and there was a trend toward the simplification of Medigap reimbursements whenever possible.

During the 1980s

The federal government first provided a *voluntary* certification option for Medigap insurers in Section 507 of the Social Security Disability Amendments of 1980 (P.L. 96-265), commonly known as the "Baucus Amendment." To meet the Baucus Amendment's *voluntary* minimum standards, the Medigap plan was required to

- meet or exceed the NAIC model standards for such plans, and
- return to policyholders as aggregate benefits at least 75% of the aggregate amount of premiums collected in group policies and at least 60% of the aggregate amount collected in individual policies.

Whether or not the insurers met these voluntary standards, the Secretary of Health, Education, and Welfare (now Health and Human Services, HHS) was required to

- make information available to Medicare beneficiaries about the value of Medigap policies,
- study the methods the states used to regulate Medigap plans, and
- report to Congress, at least once every two years, on the effectiveness of the certification procedure.

The move toward increased consumer protections was evident beginning in the late 1980s. The Medicare and Medicaid Patient and Program Protection Act of 1987 (P.L. 100-93) provided that individuals who knowingly and willfully make a false statement or misrepresent a medical fact in the sale of Medigap are guilty of a felony. The Omnibus Budget Reconciliation Act of 1987 (P.L. 100-203, OBRA87) permitted the participating physicians or suppliers to be paid directly by the Medigap plans. The Medicare Catastrophic Coverage Act of 1988 (P.L. 100-360, MCCA) improved the information available to potential Medigap purchasers by directing the Secretary of HHS to inform them about sales abuses, publish a toll-free phone number to report such abuses, and inform potential beneficiaries of the addresses and telephone numbers of state and federal offices that provide information and assistance. MCCA also *required* that Medigap plans offered in a state meet or exceed the NAIC guidelines; if this requirement was not met, federal model standards would be established for that state. Several provisions in MCAA would have made additional changes to Medicare, but they were repealed (before they went into effect) by the Medicare Catastrophic Coverage Repeal Act of 1989 (P.L. 101-234), The changes included

- expanding Medicare Part B benefits,
- imposing an annual supplemental Medicare premium on Part A beneficiaries whose tax liability equaled or exceed $150, and
- imposing an out-of-pocket maximum on Part B expenditures.

These changes would generally have lowered the Medicare beneficiary's level of cost-sharing, and therefore interact with Medigap.

During the 1990s

The Omnibus Budget Reconciliation Act of 1990 (P.L. 101-508, OBRA90) replaced some voluntary guidelines with federal standards. In particular, OBRA90

- provided for the sale of only 10 standardized Medigap plans (in all but three states);
- guaranteed plan renewability (with rare exceptions);
- prohibited the selling of policies that duplicated certain health insurance provisions to which a beneficiary was entitled, for instance through a retiree health plan;
- curtailed the use of preexisting condition limitations and other forms of health-based pricing;
- required that insurers return to policyholders as aggregate benefits at least 75% of the aggregate amount of premiums collected in group policies and at least 65% of the aggregate amount collected in individual policies; and
- introduced Medigap SELECT plans in 15 states, where SELECT plans provided a managed-care option for beneficiaries with reimbursement within a limited network.

The Act to Amend the Omnibus Budget Reconciliation Act of 1990, which was passed in 1995 (P.L. 104-18), extended the 15-state Medicare SELECT demonstration program to every state, at state option.

Two of the statutes enacted during the 1990s continued to emphasize consumer protections. The Balanced Budget Act of 1997 (P.L. 105-32,

BBA97) imposed restrictions on preexisting condition exclusions during the initial Medigap open-enrollment period when the plan purchaser is at least age 65 and meets a requirement for previous health insurance coverage. In addition, the BBA97 requested that the Secretary of HHS ask the NIAC to develop two high-deductible Medigap plans, which became known as Plan F—High Deductible Version and Plan J. The Ticket to Work and Work Incentives Improvement Act of 1999 (P.L. 106-170) permitted disabled Medicare beneficiaries to request the suspension of Medigap when they were covered under a major medical group health policy.

A few Medigap statutes passed in the 1990s primarily affected the insurance firms. The Social Security Act Amendments of 1994 (P.L. 103-432, SSAA94) modified OBRA90. As listed above, OBRA90 barred the sale of policies that duplicated other (non-Medigap) coverage to which a beneficiary was entitled. OBRA90 therefore had the unintended consequence of insurers refusing to sell Medigap policies to beneficiaries who had any other type of private coverage, however limited. SSAA94 amended the OBRA90 requirements by narrowing the anti-duplication provisions and clarifying the circumstances under which insurers could sell health insurance policies with duplicative (non-Medigap) coverage.

The Omnibus Consolidation and Emergency Supplemental Appropriation Act of 1999 (P.L. 105- 277) required that providers or facilities that paid Medigap premiums for beneficiaries be subject to civil penalties. This legislation attempted to avoid conflicts of interest created when providers or facilities first paid premiums and then self-referred patients.

During the 2000s

The Consolidated Appropriations Act, 2001 (P.L. 106-554) specified various anti-discrimination provisions. In particular, individuals who experienced certain changes in their health insurance status (e.g., involuntary termination of a Medigap plan) were guaranteed the right to purchase a new Medigap plan and were protected against preexisting conditions exclusions.

The Medicare Prescription Drug Improvement and Modernization Act of 2003 (P.L. 108-173, MMA) included various changes in Medigap plans. Because the MMA added the Medicare Part D drug provisions, Medigap plans containing drug benefits could no longer be sold to those who did not already have them. Those whose Medigap policies were issued before January 1, 2006, and did contain drug coverage were allowed to keep their existing Medigap policy as is, in some cases to keep their existing policy minus the drug benefit, or to purchase Medicare Part D together with either their old Medigap plan minus the drug benefit or certain new Medigap plans. In particular, individuals with Medigap Plan H, Plan I, and Plan J were guaranteed the right to purchase any of Plan A, Plan B, Plan C, and Plan F with the same insurance carrier. Moreover, the carrier could not use the individual's health status, claims experience, receipt of health care, or medical condition to determine the premium. Excluding preexisting conditions from these policies was also prohibited.

The MMA also requested that the Secretary of HHS request the NAIC to develop additional Medigap plans. Two plans were to incorporate coinsurance and a maximum out-of-pocket limit; no plans available in 2003 had these features. These two plans became Plan K and Plan L. Any other Medigap plans developed by the NAIC did not have to incorporate these features, but were required to exclude prescription drug benefits; Plan M and Plan N fell into this category. I n some instances, the MMA changes created two identical plans; existing Medigap Plan E, Plan H, Plan I, and Plan J were eliminated because they duplicated other plans.[11]

The Medicare Improvements for Patients and Providers Act of 2008 (P.L. 110-275, MIPPA) set standards for which plans insurers must offer. In particular, insurers who wanted to offer plans beyond the basic least comprehensive plan (Plan A) were required to offer at least one of the most comprehensive plans (Plan C or Plan F). The Genetic Information Nondiscrimination Act of 2008 (P.L. 110-343, GINA) prohibited discrimination by health insurers and employers based on genetic information. Finally, Section 3210 of the Patient Protection and Affordable Care Act of 2010 (P.L. 111-148, ACA, as amended) requested that the Secretary of HHS request that the NAIC "review and revise" cost-sharing in Plan C and Plan F.

Coordination of Payment between Medicare and Medigap

The rules governing coordination of the health insurance payments from the insurers to the Medicare service providers for services covered by Medicare Part B are mandated by Section 1842(h)(3)(B) of the Social Security Act.[12] In most cases, when a beneficiary receives care covered by Medicare Part B, the Medicare contractor pays the provider its portion of the bill. The claim is automatically forwarded to the Medigap insurer, and the Medigap insurer pays the provider its portion of the bill. Some insurers also provide this service for Medicare Part A.[13]

Plan Characteristics

This section first describes the 10 (current) standardized Medigap plans that differ in their deductibles, copayments, coinsurance, and covered services. The section then describes the nonstandard plans: prestandardized plans, older standardized plans available for renewal only, plans in states with Medigap waivers, SELECT plans, and high-deductible plans. Unless otherwise noted, the text refers to those who qualify for Medicare because they are at least age 65; Medigap options for those who qualify for Medicare because they are under age 65 and disabled are discussed later in the report.

The current standardized plans are the third generation of Medigap plans included in statue. The first group of plans predated the plan standardization mandated by OBRA90. The second group of plans (labeled Plan A through Plan J) were standardized and became effective in a state when the terms of OBRA90 were adopted by the state, which was often in 1992.

Standardized Plans

Table 2 provides information on the 10 current, standardized Medigap plans. These plans became effective on June 1, 2010, and an individual purchasing a Medigap policy for the first time (in a state without a waiver) must choose among these plans. However, not every Medigap plan is offered in each state.

These 10 plans differ with respect to generosity of benefits, cost-sharing provisions, deductibles, and other features. Plan A provides a basic set of benefits, and plan F has the most generous benefits. Plan C and Plan F cover all Medicare copayments and deductibles, and therefore provide "first dollar" or "wraparound" coverage for all covered services. [14]

Plan K and Plan L represent a move away from first dollar coverage. In addition to their outpatient copayments, these plans have "catastrophic coverage," in that once the beneficiary has exceeded an annual out-of-pocket spending limit, Medigap pays 100% of the covered costs for the remainder of the insurance year. Plan N pays 100% of the Part B coinsurance, except for a copayment of up to $20 for some office visits and up to $50 for an emergency room visit that does not result in an inpatient admission.

Table 2. Standard Medigap Plans, Effective On or After June 1, 2010

Medigap Benefits	Medigap Plans									
	A	B	C	D	F	G	K	I	M	N
Medicare Part A coinsurance and hospital costs up to an additional 365 days after Medicare benefits are used up	yes	yes	yes	yes	yes	yes	yes	yes	yes	yes
Hospice care coinsurance or copayment	yes	yes	yes	yes	yes	yes	50%	75%	yes	yes
Skilled nursing facility care coinsurance			yes	yes	yes	yes	50%	75%	yes	yes
Medicare Part A deductible		yes	yes	yes	yes	yes	50%	75%	50%	yes
Medicare Part B Coinsurance or Copayment	yes	yes	yes	yes	yes	yes	50%	75%	yes	yes (possible) copay)
Medicare Part B excess charge					yes	yes				
Medicare Part B deductible			yes		yes					
Blood	yes	yes	yes	yes	yes	yes	50%	75%	yes	yes
Foreign travel emergency (up to plan limits)			yes	yes	yes	yes			yes	yes
Out-of-pocket limit in 2012							$4,660	$2,330		

Source: Centers for Medicare & Medicaid Services, *Choosing a Medigap Policy: A Guide to Health Insurance for People with Medicare*, 2012, p. 11, http://www.medicare.gov/publications/pubs/pdf/02110.pdf and Centers for Medicare & Medicaid Services, *K & L Out-of-Pocket Limits Announcements*, September 2011, https://www.cms.gov/ Medigap/04_KandL.asp.

Notes: This table lists plans available for purchase by new Medigap enrollees as of June 1, 2010. Some of the plans had different benefits before this time. For example, the pre-June 1, 2010, Plan G contained an 80% Medicare Part B excess charge benefit and an at-home recovery benefit, while the post June 1, 2010, Plan G contained a 100% Medicare Part B excess charge benefit and no at-home recovery benefit. A "yes" in a cell indicates that Medigap covers 100% of the cost of the benefit. A percentage in a cell gives the percentage of the cost that Medigap covers. Plan K and Plan L pay 100% of covered services after the Medigap out-of-pocket limit is met. Plan N pays 100% of the Part B coinsurance, except for a copayment of up to $20 for some office visits and up to $50 for emergency room visits that do not result in an inpatient admission. Plan F is also available with a high-deductable option, where the deductible is $2,070 in 2012. Excess charges are the difference between Medicare's recognized amount and actual charges, subject to charge limitations set by Medicare and state law.

It should be noted that standardization is not absolute; rather, it serves as a national benefit floor within each plan. In each state, Medigap insurers are permitted, with the prior approval of the state insurance commissioner, to offer plans with new or innovative benefits.[15] For example, a version of Plan F offered by Regence Blue Shield of Idaho offers preventive dental benefits.[16] New or innovative benefits, however, may not be used to reduce standardized benefits.

Prestandardized Plans

Medigap plans offered before OBRA90 became effective are known as prestandardized plans. Although these plans cannot be sold to new beneficiaries, individuals who already have them may keep them. In other words, prestandardized plans are grandfathered as long as the insurer continues to offer them.

Older Standardized Plans Available for Renewal Only

Older standardized Medigap plans that were once available for purchase but are now only available for renewal are Plan E, Plan H, Plan I, and Plan J. An individual who purchased one of these plans may continue to renew his or her plan provided the insurer keeps offering the plan.[17] However, the insurer may not sell these plans to new enrollees. As with prestandardized plans, older standardized plans are grandfathered.

There is considerable variation among the benefit packages offered by these older plans. Some benefits no longer offered to new beneficiaries may be covered in these plans. For example, Plan H, Plan I, and Plan J can include drug coverage (as long as the beneficiary is not enrolled in Medicare Part D). Those who did not elect Part D may keep the drug benefits in their Medigap plans.[18] A second example of variation is the at-home recovery benefit, which is currently available in Plan D, Plan G, Plan I, and Plan J if the plans were originally sold before May 31, 2010.[19]

Medigap Plans for States with Waivers

The standardized Medigap plans do not apply to residents of Massachusetts, Minnesota, and Wisconsin.[20] These states had their own standardized Medigap plans prior to the enactment of the federal standardization requirements. The insurance carriers were permitted to continue existing state standardized plans. The states, however, were required to modify their regulatory requirements to comply with the MMA requirements (e.g., the prohibition against renewing Medigap policies with prescription drug coverage for those enrolled in Medicare Part D). The Medigap plans themselves are broadly similar to the nationally standardized plans, although they differ in their details. For example, at the time these states were granted waivers, their mandated benefits differed. In addition, Wisconsin now covers 40 visits of home health care in addition to those covered by Medicare.[21]

SELECT Plans

Medicare SELECT plans are Medigap plans that provide beneficiaries with a managed-care option with reimbursement for medical goods and services received within a limited network. Medicare SELECT is available in some states.[22] Purchasers of SELECT plans are required (except in emergencies) to obtain care through specified hospitals and, in some cases, doctors in order to have the SELECT plans pay for services rendered.[23] The beneficiaries' premiums are generally lower in SELECT plans in exchange for the restrictions in provider choice.

High-Deductible Plans

A second version of Medigap Plan F has a high deductible.[24] In a high-deductible Plan F, all copayments are paid for after the deductible is met. The premium for this plan should be less expensive than the standard (no-deductible) Plan F because a high-deductible often increases the beneficiary's out-of-pocket expenses, all else equal. The 2012 high deductible is $2,070. In addition, a second version of older Medigap Plan J is a grandfathered high-deductible plan.

Plan Enrollment

Over one-half of Medigap beneficiaries choose one of two plans. **Figure 2** provides the distribution of Medigap participants across all plans. In 2010, about 44% of beneficiaries purchased Plan F. This plan is the most comprehensive available and covers, in addition to the basic services covered in Plan A, all Medicare deductibles, copayments, and excess charges. An additional 14% of beneficiaries purchased Plan C, which includes the same benefits as Plan F, except it does not cover excess charges. In other words, the two most popular benefit plans cover all deductibles and copayments.

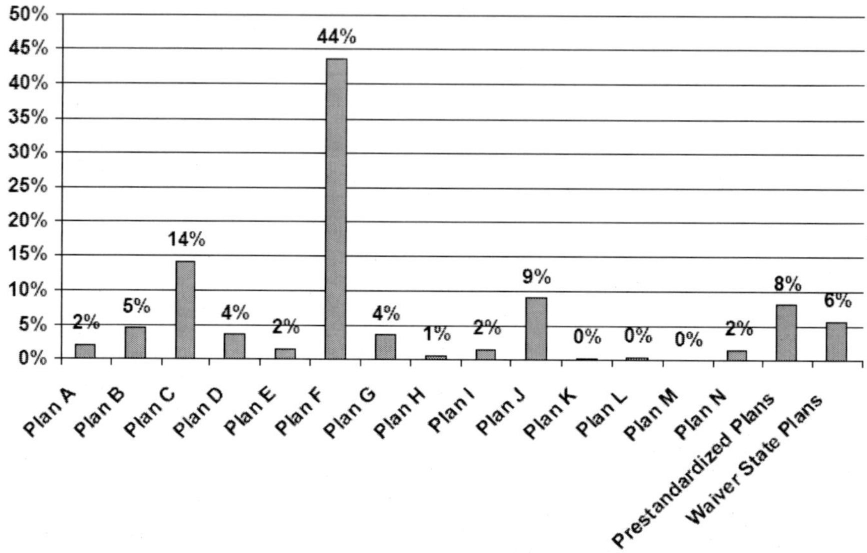

Source: Assistant Secretary for Planning and Evaluation, U.S. Department of Health and Human Services, *Variation and Trends in Medigap Premiums*, ASPE Report, December 2011, p. 15, http://aspe.hhs.gov/health/reports/ 2011/Medigap Premiums/index.shtml.The underlying data are from the NAIC.

Notes: Note that some of the plans were available for renewal only to long-time policyholders and could not be purchased by other individuals. Totals may not add to 100% because of rounding. Each state with a waiver (Massachusetts, Minnesota, and Wisconsin) offers its own standardized Medigap plans. The waiver state category also contains about 0.6% of the total number of plans that are of unknown type but are primarily issued in Illinois.

Figure 2. Distribution of Medigap Plans,All Medigap Beneficiaries, 2010.

Five plans have entered the Medigap market since 2006.[25] Sales of high-deductible Plan F, Plan K, and Plan L began in 2006, and sales of Plan M and Plan N began in 2010.These new plans have different types of cost-sharing.[26] Plan K and Plan L were the first plans to cover less than 100% of the cost of certain benefits including the Medicare Part A deductible and the Part B coinsurance and copayment. Plan K and Plan L cap out-of-pocket spending to compensate for the potentially large costs of these excluded benefits. Plan M covers 50% of the Part A deductible and does not have a cap on out-of-pocket spending. For these three plans, beneficiaries might have a relatively hard time predicting their annual costs because their costs depend on the amount and total cost of the medical services they usc. On the other hand, Plan N imposes a $20 copayment for some office visits and up to a $50 copayment for emergency room visits that do not result in an inpatient admission. Under Plan N, beneficiaries might have a relatively easier time predicting their annual costs because, while the individual's cost-sharing will vary depending on the number of visits they have, the cost-sharing does not depend on the total costs of the medical services provided. In short, Medigap plans with copayments may have more predictable costs than plans with coinsurance, all else equal. Thus plan N's cost-sharing may be more predictable than Plan K's, Plan L's, or Plan M's cost-sharing.

Because these plans are new, when looking at plan choice, it is helpful to compare their uptake across new enrollees. In other words, the following comparison looks at those choosing a policy for the first time. The individuals could choose between the plans that were available before 2006, and those which became available in 2006.

In 2011, 18% of those choosing a plan for the first time enrolled in Plan N. On the other hand, of those choosing a plan for the first time, 2% enrolled in plan K, 1% enrolled in Plan L, and less than 0.5% enrolled in Plan M.[27]

The local availability of plans may also influence the individual's choice of plan. For example, in 2011 about 36% of insurers offered Plan N, but only 17% of insurers offered Plan K, 15% of insurers offered Plan L, and 8% of insurers offered plan M.[28] It is possible that Plan N is more popular than Plan K, Plan L, and Plan M not because of the known copayments but because more insurers sell Plan N than the other three plans.[29]

Consumer Protections

This section summarizes the protections accorded to purchasers of Medigap insurance plans who are at least age 65. Consumer protections are strongest during the initial open-enrollment period and are also strong in some circumstances discussed below. The section ends with a discussion of the protections accorded to disabled beneficiaries under age 65.

During the Open-Enrollment Period

Federal law establishes an initial, one-time six-month Medigap open-enrollment period for the aged that begins on the first day of the first month the individual both is at least 65 and is enrolled in Medicare Part B.[30] Individuals are automatically enrolled in Medicare Part B at age 65.[31]

During the open-enrollment period, the individual is protected in three ways. First, insurers cannot refuse to sell the individual any Medigap policy that the insurer offers. Second, an insurer cannot set an individual's policy premiums based on the individual's health (i.e., medical underwriting). Third, insurers cannot impose a waiting period before the individual's policy can start. This third prohibition refers to the start of the entire Medigap policy and is different from a prohibition against the coverage of preexisting conditions.

For the purposes of Medigap, *preexisting conditions* are defined as those conditions diagnosed or treated during the six months immediately preceding the individual's enrollment in a Medigap policy.[32] During open enrollment, individuals may be subject to no more than a six-month preexisting exclusion period. However, preexisting condition limitations may not be imposed at all in certain cases:[33]

- If on the date of application, the individual is in the first six-month enrollment period, and has had at least six months of health insurance coverage meeting the definition of "creditable coverage" under the Health Insurance Portability and Accountability Act of 1996 (P.L. 104-191, HIPAA), he or she cannot have preexisting condition limitations. If the individual has less than six months of creditable coverage, the waiting period for the preexisting conditions is reduced by the number of months of creditable coverage.[34]
- An individual who met the exception for preexisting condition limitations in one Medigap plan does not have to meet the exception under a new plan for previously covered benefits.[35]

After the Open-Enrollment Period

If an individual applies for a Medigap policy after the open-enrollment period, the insurer is sometimes permitted to use medical underwriting. *Medical underwriting* is the use of an individual's health history to decide whether to accept the health insurance application, whether to add a waiting period for preexisting conditions (if permitted by state law), and how much to charge the individual for his or her Medigap policy.

Guaranteed Issue

Even after the open-enrollment period has passed, however, the individual may have other consumer protections when purchasing a Medigap policy in limited situations. Medigap *guaranteed issue* rights are the rights to buy a Medigap plan, have all preexisting conditions covered, and not be charged more for past or present health conditions.[36] There are four broad classes of guaranteed issue rights: rights following a change in residence or employment, rights associated with sampling a Medicare Advantage or Medicare SELECT plan (trial rights), rights triggered by certain actions by the insurer (no fault rights), and other rights.

Rights after Changes in Residence or Employment

If the individual is covered by Medicare, and his or her place of residence or labor force status changes, the individual may have guaranteed issue rights for Plan A, Plan B, Plan C, Plan F, Plan K, and Plan L. In general, to preserve these rights, the individual must apply for the Medigap plan no later than 63 calendar days after the previous health insurance coverage ends. The rights are available for the following reasons:

- An individual is enrolled in a Medicare Advantage plan and moves out of the geographic area. The individual must switch to Original Medicare before the Medigap purchase.
- An individual has Original Medicare and
  - an employer group health policy (including retiree or COBRA coverage), or
  - union coverage that is a secondary payer to Medicare, and the individual's policy ends. If the individual has COBRA coverage, guaranteed issue extends to the end of COBRA.[37] The individual may have additional rights under state law.
- An individual has Medicare SELECT and moves out of the SELECT plan's service area.

Trial Rights

Some individuals enrolled in Original Medicare may want to try out different Medicare alternatives such as Medicare Advantage or Medicare SELECT. These individuals may switch from Original Medicare to MA or Medicare SELECT, and can try out that policy for up to one year. If these individuals decide to switch back to Original Medicare within that initial year, they are guaranteed the right to enroll in a Medigap policy at that time. These rights operate as follows:

- If the individual joined MA when he or she was first eligible for Medicare Part A at age 65, within the first year of joining, the individual may switch to Original Medicare and have guaranteed issue rights for any standardized Medigap plan sold in the state.[38]
- If the individual dropped a Medigap policy to join an MA or Medicare SELECT plan for the first time, and the individual has been in the new plan for less than a year, the individual has guaranteed issue rights for the original Medigap plan if the former insurer still sells it. If the former plan is not available, the individual has guaranteed issue rights for any of Medigap Plan A, Plan B, Plan C, Plan F, Plan K, or Plan L that is sold in the state.

These rights generally last for 63 days after coverage of the forfeited MA or SELECT plan ends, although they might last for an extra 12 months under certain circumstances.

No Fault Rights

If an insurer is no longer able to sell the Medigap plan, or has not followed the requirements for Medigap insurers, or has misled the individual, the individual's purchase of Medigap Plan A, Plan B, Plan C, Plan F, Plan K, or Plan L from any insurance carrier is guaranteed as follows:[39]

- If the individual's insurer goes bankrupt or a Medigap policy ends through no fault of the individual, the individual has guaranteed issue rights.
- If the Medigap insurer commits fraud, and the individual then drops the insurer's business, the individual has guaranteed issue rights.

Other Rights

If the individual is enrolled in an MA plan and the insurer sponsoring the plan stops participating in Medicare or if the MA plan leaves the geographic area, the individual has guaranteed issue rights to purchase any of Medigap Plan A, Plan B, Plan C, Plan F, Plan K, and Plan L that is sold in the state by any insurance carrier.

The individual must be enrolled in Original Medicare before purchasing Medigap.

Guaranteed Renewal

Standardized Medigap policies are guaranteed renewable so long as the plan remains for sale in the market.[40] A Medigap insurer may only terminate a beneficiary's standardized plan if that beneficiary commits fraud, makes an untrue statement, or fails to pay the premium.

Genetic Nondiscrimination

Section 104 of the Genetic Information Nondiscrimination Act (P.L. 110-343, GINA) prohibits Medigap insurers from[41]

- using genetic information about an individual to deny coverage, adjust premiums, or impose preexisting condition exclusions;
- requiring or requesting genetic testing; and
- requesting, requiring, or purchasing genetic information for underwriting purposes.

Switching Medigap Plans

A beneficiary might want to switch Medigap plans to reduce or increase the benefit levels, change the insurance firm, or move to a less expensive plan. To purchase a new Medigap plan, the beneficiary must notify the first Medigap insurer that he or she is going to cancel that insurer's plan as of a certain date.

If the new Medigap plan starts one month before the coverage from the old Medigap plan ends, the beneficiary has 30 days to decide whether to keep the new Medigap plan.

The beneficiary must pay premiums for both the old and new Medigap plans during these thirty days.[42]

Even though a beneficiary may be able to switch Medigap plans, he or she might not want to. In particular, the consumer rights discussed above do not apply outside of the circumstances listed above.

At other times, the insurer might refuse to sell the individual a policy or increase the premium if the individual is in poor health.

Medigap for Individuals under Age 65

To be covered under Medicare before age 65, individuals must qualify for Medicare based on disability. In particular, individuals under age 65 who received cash disability benefits from Social Security or the Railroad Retirement systems for at least 24 months are entitled to Medicare Part A.[43] While there is no federal requirement that insurers sell Medigap plans to disabled individuals, some states require that Medigap plans be available to some or all of these individuals.[44] In other states, insurers choose to sell Medigap plans even though there is no requirement that they do so. If permitted by state law, insurers can use medical underwriting and charge higher premiums for the standardized plans when selling to those under age 65.

Those under age 65 covered by Medigap are entitled to all open-enrollment rights upon turning 65. Because medical underwriting is forbidden during the initial open-enrollment period, the beneficiary's premium might drop at age 65 because the beneficiary's health status can no longer affect the premium. In addition, for those who have had Medicare for at least six months immediately before turning 65, there is no preexisting condition waiting period because the beneficiaries have met the creditable coverage requirement.

Insurers' Requirements

In addition to fulfilling these consumer protection requirements, insurers must offer certain plans, set premiums for their Medigap plans, and ensure the plans return a certain amount of the dollar value of claims as benefits to the policy holders.

Required Plans

If an insurer wishes to offer any Medigap plans, the insurer must offer the basic plan (i.e., Plan A). If the insurer wishes to offer any plan(s) in addition to Plan A, the insurer must then offer at least Plan C or Plan F, before it can offer any other plan.[45]

Premiums

A *rating option* is the method by which the insurer sets premiums for health insurance policies. There are three rating options in the Medigap market. Premiums may increase over time under all three ratings options; the options differ in the conditions under which premiums may increase based on the ratings option. For example, all options allow premiums to vary with the inflation rate in the beneficiary's community, but not all options allow premiums to vary with the beneficiary's age. Depending on the state, premiums may also vary with gender, smoking status, and perhaps other variables. The three rating options are as follows:

- Under the *community rating* option, the premium does not depend on the beneficiary's age. Therefore all individuals enrolled in a particular plan pay the same premium, and it does not increase with the individual's age.
- Under the *issue-age rating* option, the premium is based on the beneficiary's age when the Medigap policy was first purchased. For example, if Plan A is sold by an insurer in Maryland for 2012, that insurer would charge a lower premium for a 65-year-old new enrollee than for a 75-year-old enrollee. However, for any given individual, the premium may not increase as the individual grows older. Premiums are therefore relatively high (when compared to premiums that are adjusted each plan year for an individual's attained age) at the time of initial purchase, but do not increase as the beneficiary ages.
- Under the *attained-age rating* option, the premium is based on the beneficiary's current (attained) age. Premiums are relatively low when the individual first purchases the policy (i.e., those who are 65), but as the individual ages, the premiums will increase.

The greatest difference between the ratings options, therefore, is the way premiums increase (or do not increase) over time. From a beneficiary's perspective, the least expensive option for any given policy at the date of purchase may not be the least expensive option over the lifetime of the policy. When comparing premiums across insurance companies, therefore, individuals need to consider the premiums (or expected premiums) over the lifetime of the policy.

Medical Loss Ratios

Definition and Rationale

The *medical loss ratio* (MLR) measures the extent to which an insurance company uses the premiums it receives to cover the claims of its beneficiaries. More precisely, the MLR is the percentage of the total premiums received that the insurance company spends on health care benefits. Thus, if a plan received $100 in premiums and spent $85 on medical claims, its MLR would be 85%. A relatively high MLR suggests that the policy holders are receiving value because they are receiving relatively more benefits, and the insurance company is retaining relatively less in administrative costs and profits. The required Medigap medical loss ratios are at least 75% for group plans and at least 65% for individual plans.[46] Should a Medigap insurer fail to meet the required ratios, the insurer is required to reimburse the beneficiaries by offering refunds or credits in order to meet the Medigap plan MLR requirement.

The required MLR is lower for individual policies than for group policies because an insurance firm's administrative costs tend to be higher for individual plans. For example, it is more expensive (per beneficiary) to market plans to individuals one at a time than it is to market to one employer (or one union or one retiree group) on behalf of multiple individuals.

Required Calculations

The actual process by which individual insurers calculate their respective MLRs involves more details and assumptions.[47] First, the insurer must calculate the MLR over the lifetime of each Medigap insurance plan (e.g., Plan A, Plan B). By assumption, the lifetime of each Medigap plan is 15 years. Second, each Medigap policy is assumed to pay out a smaller amount of premiums at the start of the policy, when the beneficiary is relatively young. Third, the insurer must have sold enough policies for the MLR calculations to be considered credible.

To illustrate the way in which the insurer calculates MLRs, consider an insurer in the individual Medigap market; this insurer must demonstrate an MLR of 65% for each plan (e.g., Plan A, Plan B). The required annual MLR, however, incorporates the anticipated changes in claims paid out over time using a benchmark. A benchmark is a standard against which the insurer's claims are assessed. The MLR for each year of the policy is compared to a benchmark loss ratio (i.e., a target value given in the *Federal Register* for that plan year).[48] In particular, each insurer first calculates the MLR (for each plan) for the policies in their first year. The MLR for these first-year plans should be at least 40%, the first year benchmark. The MLR for plans in their second year should be at least 55%, and the MLR for plans in their third year should be at least 65%. The benchmark loss ratios continue to increase until reaching 77% in the 12th year, and then stay at that level for the remainder of the 15-year period. These increasing annual MLRs will result in a cumulative medical loss-ratio of at least 65%. An insurer who has met these annual benchmarks for a plan has satisfied the MLR criteria for that plan. To be in compliance with the statute, the insurer needs to meet the MLR for all the plans it offers.

In addition, insurers are permitted to apply a credibility adjustment to the MLR calculation. If there are not a sufficiently large number of policies written, the estimates and calculations are assumed to have less credibility, and the calculated MLR is permitted to be lower before the insurer is required to offer refunds or credits. In the extreme, a policy loss ratio based on less than 500 life-years since its inception is considered not credible, because there are not enough life-years observed to evaluate the actions of the insurer. In this case, no refund or credit by the insurer is required. The MLR in the group market is calculated the same way, but the loss ratio benchmarks are higher in each year because the statutory MLR is 75% and not 65%.[49]

The Role of the National Association of Insurance Commissioners

The National Association of Insurance Commissioners (NAIC) is an association of insurance regulators from the 50 states, Washington, DC, and four U.S. territories.[50]

One of the Association's stated goals is to make state regulation more consistent and uniform.[51] The NAIC also collects financial information from insurance companies; some of the data presented in this report were collected by the NAIC.[52]

The specific provisions (e.g., levels of cost-sharing and types of coverage) of all Medigap plans (excluding those in waiver states) are formulated by the NAIC. Once finalized, the standardized plans are known as *NAIC model standards* for Medigap plans.

The NAIC, however, has no authority to monitor whether the states comply with its model standards. Instead, states retain regulatory authority. States must either

- adopt the NAIC model standards and any subsequent revisions, or
- enact regulatory provisions that are more stringent that those in the NAIC model standards or in the regulatory requirements.[53]

If a states fails to adopt the NAIC model standards, the state will be considered out of compliance with federal requirements and will not be permitted to regulate its Medigap market.[54] In this case, the Centers for Medicare & Medicaid Services of HHS would regulate the sale of Medigap plans.

The NAIC has been actively involved in the evolution of the standardized Medigap plans. Changes are made over time to reflect changing health care statutes and practices. For example, a Medigap "preventive care" benefit was eliminated in 2010 because expanded Medicare Part B benefits made the Medigap preventive care benefit unnecessary. More recently, Section 3210 of ACA requests that the Secretary of HHS ask the NAIC to "review and revise" cost-sharing in two Medigap plans.

Descriptions of Medigap Markets

This section discusses Medigap premiums, the number of insurance firms in each Medigap market (known as market concentration), the level of participation in Medigap across states, and the socio-demographic characteristics of the Medigap beneficiaries. Because Medigap is sold and regulated by states, each state is its own Medigap market.

Medigap Premiums and Plan Choice

Medigap premiums for the same exact standardized plan (e.g., Plan F) may not be the same across any or all insurers offering that plan in a state. In fact, there is wide variation in Medigap premiums for each plan nationwide. For example, according to one study, the average monthly premium for Medigap Plan F in 2010 was $193 in Maryland, $149 in Virginia, and $170 in Washington, DC.[55]

This variation reflects the geographic variations in the price levels, state regulations, smoking, gender, and possibly other discounts, and the rating structure used. Even controlling for these differences, however, variations in premiums remain. [56] Individuals do not always purchase the least expensive version of their chosen plan. There are a number of hypotheses concerning this behavior: [57]

- Many of the price comparisons are available on the Internet (at the state insurance websites), and some of the elderly are not Internet-savvy.
- There may be cognitive impairment in this age group, and the large number of choices associated with selecting a Medigap plan could prove daunting.
- Potential Medigap beneficiaries may prefer to remain with their existing (pre-Medicare) insurance agent, even though the existing agent may not sell what would be the best plans for these beneficiaries.
- Certain insurers attract individuals through name recognition.[58]

Medigap Market Participation by Individuals Across States

Figure 3 provides the number of Medigap enrollees in 2010 by state. Enrollment varies from a low of 4,221 individuals in Hawaii to a high of 643,156 individuals in Florida. Other states with a high Medigap enrollment include Texas, Pennsylvania, and Illinois. Figure 3 is informative from a financial perspective in that it indicates which states have relatively more dollars in the Medigap market. However, the map does not provide any information about whether Ohio has a higher Medigap enrollment than North Dakota because a larger number of those eligible for Medigap actually enroll, or simply because Ohio has more residents than North Dakota.

Figure 4 shows the percentage of those enrolled in Medicare who purchase Medigap plans, and presents a different picture than **Figure 3**. The percentage of those enrolled in Medicare who purchase Medigap plans is relatively high in parts of the Midwest and mountain states and relatively low in the Southwest. That Medigap policies are popular in the Midwest is consistent with the Medicare Advantage data. In 2011, the participation rate in Medicare Advantage was lower in the Midwest and mountain states than in many other areas of the country.[59] In short, participation is Medicare Advantage is relatively lower in those states where participation in Medigap is relatively high.

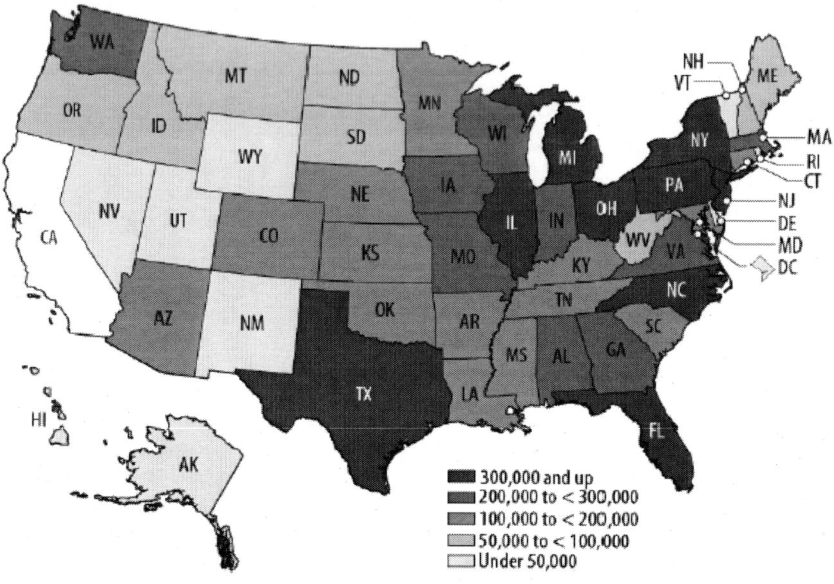

Source: Created by CRS, based on the NAIC data contained in America's Health Insurance Plans, *Trends in Medigap Coverage and Enrollment, 2010-2011*, July 2011, pp. A1-A3, http://www.ahipresearch.org/pdfs/ Medigap2011.pdf.

Notes: Complete data for California are not available. California has both a Department of Insurance and a Department of Managed Care. These two departments are governed by different regulations, and only the former is required to file data with the NAIC. More information on the Department of Insurance is available at http://insurance.ca.gov. More information on the Department of Managed Care is available at http://www.dmhc.ca.gov.

Figure 3. Medigap Enrollment, by State, 2010.

Medigap Markets by Characteristics of Enrollees

Limited public information is available on the socio-economic characteristics of those individuals who participate in Medigap. The information reported here comes from various components and years of the Medicare Current Beneficiary Survey. In broad terms, the conclusions across the three studies discussed below are consistent.

A report by America's Health Insurance Plans (AHIP, a trade group) emphasized the differences in take-up rates and socio-economic characteristics between rural and urban beneficiaries in 2010.[60] AHIP concluded that 31% of

Medigap beneficiaries lived in rural areas, while only 24% of all Medicare beneficiaries did so. AHIP also observed Medigap holders in rural areas were more likely to have lower incomes than their urban peers.

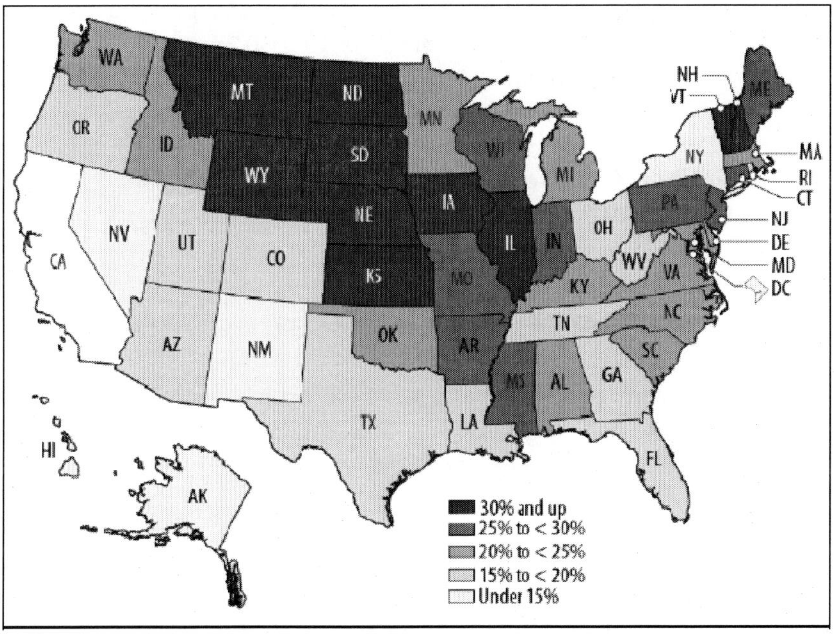

Source: CRS calculations using two data sources. The total Medicare data cover July 2010 and are from Table 2.8 of the Medicare & Medicaid Statistical Supplement, https://www.cms.gov/MedicareMedicaidStatSupp/ 08_2011.asp#TopOfPage. The Medigap data cover December 2010, and are based on NAIC data contained in America's Health Insurance Plans, *Trends in Medigap Coverage and Enrollment, 2010-2011*, July 2011, pp. A1-A3, http://www.ahipresearch.org/pdfs/ Medigap2011.pdf.

Note: Complete data for California are not available. California has both a Department of Insurance and a Department of Managed Care. These two departments are governed by different regulations, and only the former is required to file data with the NAIC. More information on the Department of Insurance is available at http://insurance.ca.gov. More information on the Department of Managed Care is available at http://www.dmhc.ca.gov.

Figure 4. Percent of Medicare Enrollees with Medigap Coverage, by State, 2010.

Comprehensive 2007 data are found in the chart pack published by The Henry J. Kaiser Family Foundation.[61] An evaluation of socio-economic characteristics showed that, of those with incomes of $10,000 or less, 7% were covered by Medigap, 7% were covered by employer-sponsored insurance, and 51% were covered by Medicaid. Of those in (self-reported) poor health, 11% were covered by Medigap, but of those in excellent or very good health, 24% were covered by Medigap. Individuals with cognitive impairments were more likely to be covered by Medicaid, and less likely to be covered by either Medigap or employer-sponsored insurance.

Finally, the Medicare Payment Advisory Commission (MedPAC) reported broadly similar results for 2007. Of poor individuals, 13% were covered by Medigap, 9% were covered by employer-sponsored insurance, and 46% were covered by Medicaid. Of those in poor health, 17% were covered by Medigap, but of those in excellent or very good health, 28% were covered by Medigap.[62]

Current Policy Issues

The focus of current policy issues has been on proposed changes to the Medigap MLR and cost-sharing levels. Background information on these topics was provided above, and current issues are discussed below.

Increasing Medical Loss Ratios

Companion bills introduced in the 112th Congress, H.R. 2645 and S. 1416, the Medigap Medical Loss Ratio Improvement Act of 2011, seek to increase the medical loss ratio required of Medigap insurers. Currently, comprehensive and major medical health insurance policies (not Medigap policies) sold in the large group market are required to have an 85% MLR, and those sold in the small group and individual markets are required to have an 80% MLR. Insurers who fail to meet these standards must provide rebates to their customers.[63]

Medigap plans have a 75% MLR requirement for the group market and a 65% MLR requirement for the individual market. In other words, private major medical and comprehensive insurers must return more of the premiums received to their beneficiaries than Medigap insurers must return to their beneficiaries. AARP and others have lobbied for an increase in the Medigap MLRs to the levels found in the comprehensive and major medical health insurance market.[64]

Those in favor of increasing MLRs argue that Medigap enrollees should have the same protections as enrollees of other private health insurance policies. In other words, a low MLR suggests that insurers keep more of claim dollars instead of returning them as benefits. Those opposed to the change argue that Medigap plans have lower premium bases over which to spread administrative costs, and therefore should be allowed to retain greater a share of premiums.[65]

Increasing Cost-Sharing

Section 3210 of the ACA requires the Secretary of HHS to request the NAIC to "review and revise" the Medigap benefit packages in order to encourage nominal cost-sharing under Plan C and Plan F. Similarly, President Obama's FY2013 budget proposal would provide incentives to increase cost-sharing. Beginning in 2017, the proposal would impose a Part B premium surcharge for new Medicare beneficiaries who select a Medigap plan with low cost-sharing requirements (i.e., offer "near first-dollar" coverage). The surcharge would be equal to approximately 15% of the average Medigap premium. This is equivalent to about 30% of the Part B premium. Moreover, the June 2012 MedPAC Report to the Congress also recommends a new charge for Medigap policies as part of a series of Medicare reforms.[66]

Cost-sharing, by requiring the beneficiary to pay more for some medical care, is often thought to discourage the beneficiary's demand for excessive health services.[67] If this is true, an increase in Medigap cost-sharing might lead to a decrease in medical goods and services used by the beneficiary, and therefore a decrease in Medicare expenditures and the federal deficit.

Some early evidence that an increase in cost-sharing leads to decrease in expenditures was provided by the RAND Health Insurance Experiment (HIE).[68] The HIE randomly assigned individuals under age 65 to "treatments" of various levels of cost-sharing. The HIE evaluation concluded that for every 10% the cost of medical services to the family increased, the family's use of medical services would fall by 2%.

The population of special interest for Medigap is largely individuals aged 65 and over who would experience an increase in cost-sharing for the health insurance policy. These individuals may respond differently than younger adults to changes in cost-sharing for a variety of reasons, including lower and/or fixed incomes, lower levels of health, and uncertainty about their lifespan. Nevertheless, the RAND result has also held up among samples of older individuals, even though the RAND experiment did not include individuals over age 64 and was conducted about 30 years ago.[69]

Two additional recent studies conclude that increased financial responsibility reduces medical care use among the elderly, but also illustrate some of the dangers of oversimplifying this matter. One study compared individuals across a staggered set of copayment changes faced by those receiving supplemental health insurance from the California Public Employees Retirement system. The researchers estimated physician visits and prescription drug utilization were "modestly price sensitive" among the elderly.[70] The second study looked at the effects of increased copayments on ambulatory care over time. When their copayments doubled, elderly individuals, when compared with a control group, had almost 20 fewer annual outpatient visits per 100 individuals.[71] However, the cost-sharing issue is more complicated than the above discussion suggests. In the first study, as the individuals reduced their physician visits and prescription drug utilization, the most ill individuals also increased their hospital utilization.[72] In the second study, individuals with increased copayments were sometimes found to have worse health outcomes and an increased total spending on health care.[73] A more complete picture of cost-sharing therefore suggests that increasing copayments can reduce health status among certain populations and ultimately increase health care spending among these populations.[74]

End Notes

[1] Medigap is also known as *Medicare Supplement* Insurance. Cost-sharing refers to the amount paid by the individual for Medicare-allowable goods and services (excluding premiums). Cost-sharing includes a *deductible*, or a set dollar amount the beneficiary must pay before Medicare provides any reimbursement for most services. Cost-sharing also includes *copayments* and/or *coinsurance*, with Medicare paying the remaining (allowable) costs. In general usage, copayment refers to a flat amount (e.g., $30 per visit), whereas coinsurance refers to a percentage (e.g., 20% of the total visit charge).

[2] Most beneficiaries enrolled in Medicare Advantage can only receive prescription drugs through their plan. Only those enrolled in a Medicare Private Fee-for-Service MA plan may purchase a stand-alone Part D prescription drug plan.

[3] Most individuals do not pay a premium for Part A because they or their spouses paid at least 40 quarters of Medicare payroll taxes while working.

[4] Home health services, community health services, some preventive services, and some other services are not subject to the Part B deductible.

[5] For more information on Medicare, see CRS Report R40425, *Medicare Primer*, coordinated by Patricia A. Davis.

[6] If an individual purchased a Medigap plan prior to enrolling in MA, he or she may continue to enroll in the Medigap plan. The Medigap plan, however, cannot cover deductibles, copayments, coinsurance, or premiums under the MA plan. For more information, see

Centers for Medicare & Medicaid Services, *Medicare and You*, 2012, p. 68, http://www.medicare.gov/publications/pubs/pdf/10050.pdf.

[7] This report cites studies that generally use one of two data sources. The first data source is the National Association of Insurance Commissioners (NAIC). The NAIC is an association of insurance regulators from the 50 states, Washington, DC, and four U.S. territories. The NAIC collects financial information from insurance companies. Data collected by the NAIC is administrative data, and provides relatively more detailed information on the characteristics of Medigap plans sold. The second data source is the Access to Care file of the Medicare Current Beneficiary Survey (MCBS), which includes self-reported data on whether an individual holds a Medigap plan. The survey data provides relatively more detailed information on the characteristics of the Medigap plan beneficiaries. These two data sources are not necessarily comparable.

Moreover, estimates from different organizations may not be comparable even when the same data source is used. For example, both the Kaiser Family Foundation and the Office of the Assistant Secretary for Policy Evaluation (ASPE) of the Department of Health and Human Services use data from the Access to Care file of the MCBS, but the organizations' estimates are not comparable. At a minimum, these organizations define variables slightly differently, and differ in their treatment of missing values.

[8] *Medicaid* is a means-tested individual entitlement program that finances the delivery of primary care medical services, acute care medical services, and long-term care services and supports. Within broad federal guidelines, each state designs and administers its own program.

[9] A group health policy is defined in Section 5000(a)(1) of the Internal Revenue Code to mean "a plan (including a self-insured plan) of, or contributed to by, an employer (including a self-employed person) or employee organization to provide health care (directly or otherwise) to the employees, former employees, the employer, others associated or formerly associated with the employer in a business relationship, or their families."

[10] For information on the federal regulation of pension plans, health plans, and other employee benefit plans, see archived CRS Report RL34443, *Summary of the Employee Retirement Income Security Act (ERISA)*, by Patrick Purcell and Jennifer Staman.

[11] Centers for Medicare & Medicaid Services, "Medicare Program: Recognition of NAIC Model Standards for Regulation of Medicare Supplemental Insurance," 74 *Federal Register* 18810, April 24, 2009.

[12] No comparable statute exists for Part A.

[13] Centers for Medicare & Medicaid Services, *Choosing a Medigap Policy: A Guide to Health Insurance for People with Medicare*, 2012, p. 20, http://www.medicare.gov/publications/pubs/pdf/02110.pdf.

[14] First dollar coverage of a good or service means that the insurance plan covers 100% of the cost of the good or service (up to any maximum). All plans have first-dollar coverage for preventive care and certain other services.

[15] 74 *Federal Register* 18823.

[16] Regence BlueShield of Idaho, "Regence Bridge Medigap (Medicare Supplement) Plans," p. 8, http://www.regence.com/docs/ID/medicare2011/medigap-sales-brochure.pdf.

[17] Centers for Medicare & Medicaid Services, "Medicare Program: Recognition of NAIC Model Standards for Regulation of Medicare Supplemental Insurance," 74 *Federal Register* 18825, April 24, 2009.

[18] For information on the conditions under which Medigap with drug benefits and Part D could be exchanged, see Center for Medicare & Medicaid Services, *Your Guide to Medicare*

Prescription Drug Coverage, revised May 2009, pp. 37-54, http://www.medicare.gov/ Publications/Pubs/pdf/11109.pdf.

[19] Medicare Interactive, http://www.medicarerights.org/pdf/Pre-2010Medigap-Benefits-National-2012update.pdf.

[20] 74 *Federal Register* 18809.

[21] Center for Medicare & Medicaid Services, *2012 Choosing a Medigap Policy: A Guide to Health Insurance for People with Medicare*, December 2011, pp. 42-44, http://www.medicare.gov/Publications/Pubs/pdf/02110.pdf, and Center for Medicare & Medicaid Services, *Medicare and Home Health Care*, May 2010, http://www.medicare.gov/ publications/pubs/pdf/10969.pdf.

[22] 74 *Federal Register* 18823. The insurance contracts for these *Medigap* plans are known as *Medicare* SELECT.

[23] Medicare always pays its share for services whether or not the provider is a SELECT provider.

[24] 74 *Federal Register* 18809.

[25] The five plans are Plan K and Plan L (whose development by NAIC was requested by the MMA), high-deductible Plan F (which was described in the BBA97), and Plan M and Plan N,

[26] All information in this paragraph is from American's Health Insurance Plans, *Trends in Medigap Coverage and Enrollment, 2011*, May 2012. Information on high-deductible Plan F was collected in a different and less reliable way than information on the other plans.

[27] The high-deductible version of plan F was chosen by between 1% and 3% of new enrollees.

[28] American's Health Insurance Plans, *Trends in Medigap Coverage and Enrollment, 2010-2011*, July 2011, p. 4, http://www.ahipresearch.org/pdfs/Medigap2011.pdf.

[29] If not all insurers offered Plan L or Plan M and if the insurers learned that individuals purchased these plans, when offered, some additional insurers might begin offering them.

[30] 74 *Federal Register* 18825.

[31] Individuals who are covered by employer-sponsored health insurance (ESI), based on either their own on their spouse's active employment, when they turn 65, however, may delay purchasing Part B at that time because they would have to pay a premium for benefits that are (usually) already covered by ESI. The six-month Medigap open-enrollment period for these individuals begins when they purchase Part B, usually when they are no longer covered through ESI based on active employment. Some states have additional open-enrollment periods.

[32] 74 *Federal Register* 18818.

[33] Broad limits on the use by insurers of preexisting conditions were imposed by the Health Insurance Portability and Accountability Act of 1996 (P.L. 104-191, HIPAA).

[34] The insurer may impose a preexisting exclusion limitation if the individual did not have such creditable coverage. Creditable coverage generally requires that there has not been a break in health insurance coverage for more than 63 days.

[35] An insurer could impose exclusions for newly covered benefits.

[36] 74 *Federal Register* 18825-18826.

[37] COBRA coverage takes its name from the Consolidated Omnibus Budget Reconciliation Act of 1985 (P.L. 99-272). COBRA requires employers with 20 or more employees to provide employees and their families the right to continue participation in the employer's group health policy in case of certain events, one of which is involuntary dismissal. For more information on COBRA, see CRS Report R40142, *Health Insurance Continuation Coverage Under COBRA*, by Janet Kinzer.

[38] The guaranteed issue right also holds if the individual joins the Programs of All-Inclusive Care For the Elderly (PACE). PACE is a capitated benefit permanently authorized by the BBA97 with a comprehensive service delivery system and integrated Medicare and Medicaid financing.

[39] 74 *Federal Register* 18826.

[40] 74 *Federal Register* 18818.

[41] For additional information on GINA, see CRS Report RL34584, *The Genetic Information Nondiscrimination Act of 2008 (GINA)*, by Amanda K. Sarata and James V. DeBergh.

[42] Centers for Medicare & Medicaid Services, *Choosing a Medigap Policy: A Guide to Health Insurance for People with Medicare*, 2012, pp. 32-35, http://www.medicare.gov/publications/pubs/pdf/02110.pdf.

[43] Centers for Medicare & Medicaid Services, *Choosing a Medigap Policy: A Guide to Health Insurance for People with Medicare*, 2011, p. 39-40, http://www.medicare.gov/publications/pubs/pdf/02110.pdf. Many disabilities qualify. In addition, a few specific illnesses/diseases have special provisions for Medicare enrollment; examples include End-Stage Renal Disease (ESRD, or permanent kidney failure requiring dialysis or a kidney transplant) and Amyotrophic Lateral Sclerosis (ALS, also known as Lou Gehrig's disease).

[44] 74 *Federal Register* 18829.

[45] 74 *Federal Register* 18823. See also Centers for Medicare & Medicaid Services, *Choosing a Medigap Policy: A Guide to Health Insurance for People with Medicare*, 2012, p. 12, http://www.medicare.gov/publications/pubs/pdf/ 02110.pdf.

[46] In this context, policies issued as a result of the solicitation of individuals through mail or by mass media advertising are considered individual policies.

[47] U.S. General Accounting Office (now called the Government Accountability Office), *Medigap Insurance: Compliance With Federal Standards Has Increased*, HEHS-98-66, March 1998, http://www.gao.gov/archive/1998/ he98066.pdf.

[48] 74 *Federal Register* 18872-18875.

[49] 74 *Federal Register* 18829. The MLR statutes are found at SSA, Section 1882(r).

[50] More formally, the NAIC is a private Internal Revenue Code section 501(c)(3) nonprofit association. The NAIC members are the elected or appointed state government officials who, along with their departments and staff, regulate the conduct of insurance companies and agents in their respective state or territory.

[51] For additional goals, see *About the NAIC*, NAIC, http://www.naic.org/index_about.htm.

[52] In some states, not all insurers report to the state insurance commissions and therefore not all insurers report to the NAIC. For example, health insurance issuers regulated by California's Department of Managed Health Care are not required by state regulators to submit data to the NAIC.

[53] 74 *Federal Register* 18809.

[54] Implementation Materials for Revisions to Medigap Model, NAIC, http://www.naic.org/documents/committees_b_senior_issues_medigap_impl_guide.pdf, p.1.

[55] Gretchen Jacobson, Tricia Neuman, and Thomas Rice, et al., *Medigap Reform: Setting the Context*, Kaiser Family Foundation, Issue Brief, September 2011, p. 7, http://www.kff.org/medicare/upload/8235-2.pdf.

[56] Nicole Maestas, Mathis Schroeder, and Dana Goldman, *Price Variation in Markets with Homogeneous Goods: The Case of Medigap*, NBER, Working Paper 14679, January 2009, pp. 1-6, http://www.nber.org/papers/w14679.

[57] *Ibid.*

[58] For example, most individuals have heard of the Blue Cross/Blue Shield insurers. In addition, many individual policies are purchased in conjunction with the AARP. Individuals who contact the AARP about Medigap are referred to United Healthcare and may then go on to purchase individual Medigap policies from this insurance firm. The AARP markets the plans while United Healthcare is the insurer who bears the risk associated with that insurance. At the national level, United had a national market share of about 46% between 2004 and 2008; see Amanda Starc, *Insurer Pricing and Consumer Welfare: Evidence from Medigap*, Harvard Business School, Working Paper, November 29, 2010, pp 5-9 for details..

[59] The Henry J. Kaiser Family Foundation, *Medicare: Medicare Advantage*, Fact Sheet, November 2011, p. 1, http://www.kff.org/medicare/upload/2052-15.pdf.

[60] America's Health Insurance Plans, *Low-Income & Rural Beneficiaries with Medigap Coverage, 2010*, May 2012, http://www.ahipresearch.org/MedigapLow IncomeRural Report2012.pdf. The underlying data come from the Medicare Current Beneficiary Survey.

[61] Juliette Cubanski, Tricia Neuman, and Anthony Damico, et al., Examining Sources of Supplemental Insurance and Prescription Drug Coverage Among Medicare Beneficiaries: Findings from the Medicare Current Beneficiary Survey, 2007, The Henry J. Kaiser Family Foundation, August 2009, pp. 2-3, http://www.kff.org/medicare/upload/7801-02.pdf. Individuals with employer-sponsored coverage were categorized as employer-sponsored, even if the individuals also carried Medigap.

[62] MedPAC, *Healthcare Spending and the Medicare Program*, June 2011, p. 54, http://www.medpac.gov/documents/ Jun11DataBookEntireReport.pdf.

[63] CRS Report R41439, *Health Insurance Agents and Brokers in the Reformed Health Insurance Market*, by Bernadette Fernandez.

[64] Dena Bunis, "Democrats Want New MLR Standards to Apply To Medigap Policies," *CQ Healthbeat News*, July 26, 2011, http://www.cq.com/doc/hbnews-3916554?wr=RDlYTlRja3lSajV1TVYqOXdwRDVWdw. AARP is usually seen as an advocate for senior citizens.

[65] Ibid.

[66] MedPAC, *Medicare and the Health Care Delivery System*, Report to the Congress, June 2012, p. 4, http://www.medpac.gov/documents/jun11_entirereport.pdf,

[67] Willard G. Manning, Joseph P. Newhouse, and Naihua Duan, et al., "Health Insurance and the Demand for Medical Care: Evidence from a Randomized Experiment," *American Economic Review*, vol. 77, no. 3 (June 1987), pp. 251-277.

[68] Willard G. Manning, Joseph P. Newhouse, and Naihua Duan, et al., "Health Insurance and the Demand for Medical Care: Evidence from a Randomized Experiment," *American Economic Review*, vol. 77, no. 3 (June 1987), pp. 251-277.

[69] Katherine Baicker and Dana Goldman, "Patient Cost-Sharing and Healthcare Spending Growth," *Journal of Economic Perspectives*, vol. 25, no. 2 (Spring 2011), p. 55.

[70] Amitabh Chandra, Jonathan Gruber, and Robin McKnight, "Patient Cost-Sharing and Hospitalization Offsets in the Elderly," *American Economic Review* , vol. 100, no. 1 (March 2010), p. 194.

[71] Amal N. Trivedi, Husein Moloo, and Vincent Mor, "Increased Ambulatory Care Copayments and Hospitalizations among the Elderly," *The New England Journal of Medicine*, vol. 362, no. 4 (January 28, 2010), p. 320.

[72] Amitabh Chandra, Jonathan Gruber, and Robin McKnight, "Patient Cost-Sharing and Hospitalization Offsets in the Elderly," *American Economic Review*, vol. 100, no. 1 (March 2010), p. 194.

[73] Amal N. Trivedi, Husein Moloo, and Vincent Mor, "Increased Ambulatory Care Copayments and Hospitalizations among the Elderly," *The New England Journal of Medicine*, vol. 362, no. 4 (January 28, 2010), p. 320.

[74] Katherine Swartz, *Cost-Sharing: Effects on Spending and Outcomes*, Robert Wood Johnson Foundation, Research Synthesis Report No. 20, December 2010, pp. 1-5, http://www.rwjf.org/files/research/ 121710.policysynthesis.costsharing.rpt.pdf, and Robert Wood Johnson Foundation, *Cost-Sharing: Effects on Spending and Outcomes*, Policy Brief, December 2010, p. 1, http://www.rwjf.org/files/research/ 121710.policysynthesis.cost sharing.brief.pdf.

In: Medigap
Editor: Johny P. Hughes

ISBN: 978-1-62417-279-3

Chapter 2

Choosing a Medigap Policy: A Guide to Health Insurance for People with Medicare*

U.S. Department of Health and Human Services

This offcial government guide has important information about the following:

- What is a Medigap (Medicare Supplement Insurance) policy
- What Medigap policies cover
- Your rights to buy a Medigap policy
- How to buy a Medigap policy

This guide can help if you're thinking about buying a Medigap policy or already have one.

Who Should Read This Guide?

This guide helps people with Medicare understand Medigap (also called "Medicare Supplement Insurance") policies. A Medigap policy is a type of

* This is an edited, reformatted and augmented version of U.S. Department of Health and Human Services.

private insurance that helps you pay for some of the costs that Original Medicare doesn't cover.

Section 1. Medicare Basics

A Brief Look at Medicare

This guide helps people with Medicare understand Medigap (also called "Medicare Supplement Insurance") policies.

A Medigap policy is health insurance sold by private insurance companies to fill gaps in Original Medicare coverage. Medigap policies can help pay your share (coinsurance, copayments, or deductibles) of the costs of Medicare-covered services. Some Medigap policies also cover certain benefits Original Medicare doesn't cover. Medigap policies don't cover your share of the costs under other types of health coverage, including Medicare Advantage Plans, stand-alone Medicare Prescription Drug Plans, employer/union group health coverage, Medicaid, Department of Veterans Affairs (VA) benefits, or TRICARE. Insurance companies generally can't sell you a Medigap policy if you have coverage through Medicaid or a Medicare Advantage Plan.

Before you learn more about Medigap policies, the next few pages provide a brief look at Medicare. If you already know the basics about Medicare and only want to learn about Medigap, skip to Section 2: Medigap Basics.

What is Medicare?

Medicare is health insurance for the following:

- People 65 or older
- People under 65 with certain disabilities
- People of any age with End-Stage Renal Disease (ESRD) (permanent kidney failure requiring dialysis or a kidney transplant)

The Different Parts of Medicare

The different parts of Medicare help cover specific services:

Medicare Part A (Hospital Insurance)
• Helps cover inpatient care in hospitals • Helps cover skilled nursing facility, hospice, and home health care
Medicare Part B (Medical Insurance)
• Helps cover doctors' and other health care providers' services, hospital outpatient care, durable medical equipment, and home health care • Helps cover many preventive servicesto help maintain your health and to keep certain illnesses from getting worse
Medicare Part C (also known as Medicare Advantage)
Offers health plan options run by Medicare-approved private insurance companies. Medicare Advantage Plansare a way to get the benefits and services covered under Part A and Part B. Most Medicare Advantage Plans cover Medicare prescription drugcoverage (Part D). Some Medicare Advantage Plans may include extra benefits for an extra cost.
Medicare Part D (Medicare Prescription Drug Coverage)
• Helps cover the cost of prescription drugs • May help lower your prescription drug costs and help protect against higher costs • Run by Medicare-approved private insurance companies

Your Medicare Coverage Choices at a Glance

There are two main ways to get your Medicare coverage: Original Medicare or a Medicare Advantage Plan. Use these steps to help you decide which way to get your coverage. See Section 5 for information about Medicare Advantage Plans and Medigap policies.

For More Information

Remember, this guide is about Medigap policies. To learn more about Medicare, visit www.medicare.gov/publications to view the "Medicare & You" handbook. You can also call 1-800-MEDICARE (1-800-633-4227). TTY users should call 1-877-486-2048.

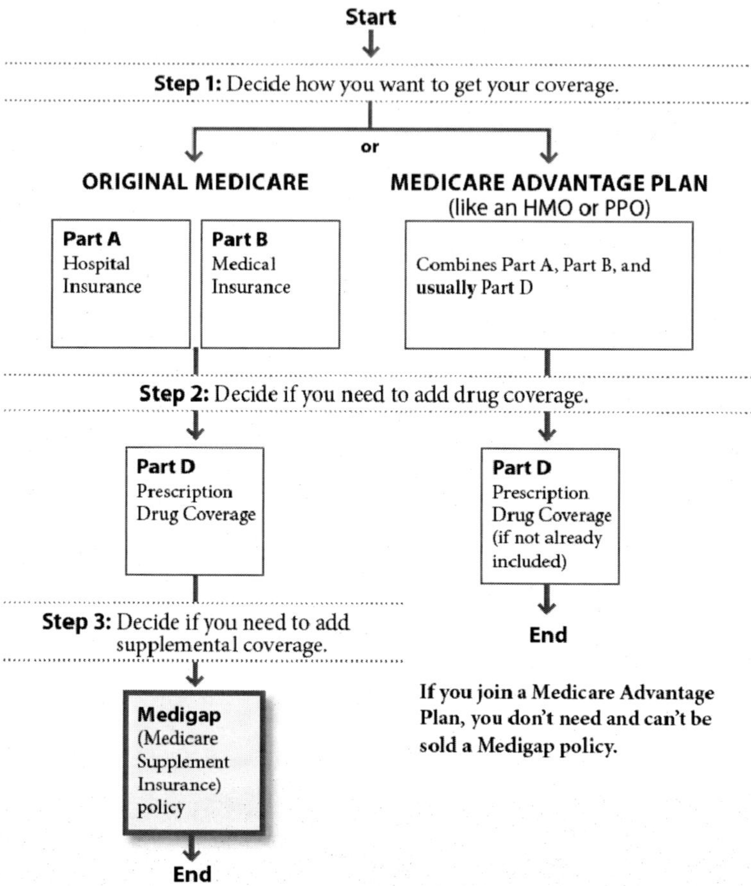

Section 2. Medigap Basics

What is a Medigap Policy?

A Medigap policy (also called "Medicare Supplement Insurance") is private health insurance that's designed to supplement Original Medicare. This means it helps pay some of the health care costs ("gaps") that Original Medicare doesn't cover (like copayments, coinsurance, and deductibles). If you have Original Medicare and a Medigap policy, Medicare will pay its share of the Medicare-approved amounts for covered health care costs. Then your

Medigap policy pays its share. A Medigap policy is different from a Medicare Advantage Plan (like an HMO or PPO) because those plans are ways to get Medicare benefits, while a Medigap policy only supplements your Original Medicare benefits.

Note: Medicare doesn't pay any of the costs for you to get a Medigap policy.

Every Medigap policy must follow Federal and state laws designed to protect you, and the policy must be clearly identified as "Medicare Supplement Insurance." Medigap insurance companies in most states can only sell you a "standardized" Medigap policy identified by letters A through N. Each standardized Medigap policy must offer the same basic benefits, no matter which insurance company sells it. Cost is usually the only difference between Medigap policies with the same letter sold by different insurance companies. In Massachusetts, Minnesota, and Wisconsin, Medigap policies are standardized in a different way. See Section 7. In some states, you may be able to buy another type of Medigap policy called Medicare SELECT. SELECT plans are standardized plans that may require you to see certain providers and may cost less than other plans. See Section 2.

What Medigap Policies Cover

The Medigap Plans chart gives you a quick look at the standardized Medigap Plans available.

Note:

- Insurance companies selling Medigap policies are required to make Plan A available. If they offer any other Medigap plan, they must also offer either Medigap Plan C or Plan F. Not all types of Medigap policies may be available in your state. See Section 7 if you live in **Massachusetts**, **Minnesota**, or **Wisconsin**. If you need more information, call your State Insurance Department or State Health Insurance Assistance Program. See Section 8 for your state's phone number.
- **Plans D and G** —Plans D and G effective on or after June 1, 2010, have different benefits than D or G Plans bought before June 1, 2010.
- **Plans No Longer for Sale** —Plans E, H, I, and J are no longer sold, **but**, if you already have one, you can keep it.

Medigap Plans

How to read the chart:

If a check mark appears in a column of this chart, the Medigap policy covers 100% of the described benefit. If a row lists a percentage, the policy covers that percentage of the described benefit. If a row is blank, the policy doesn't cover that benefit. **Note:** The Medigap policy covers coinsurance only after you have paid the deductible (unless the Medigap policy also covers the deductible).

Medigap Benefits	A	B	C	D	F*	G	K	L	M	N
Medicare Part A Coinsurance and hospital costs up to an additional 365 days after Medicare benefits are used up	✓	✓	✓	✓	✓	✓	✓	✓	✓	✓
Medicare Part B Coinsurance or Copayment	✓	✓	✓	✓	✓	✓	50%	75%	✓	✓***
Blood (First 3 Pints)	✓	✓	✓	✓	✓	✓	50%	75%	✓	✓
Part A Hospice Care Coinsurance or Copayment	✓	✓	✓	✓	✓	✓	50%	75%	✓	✓
Skilled Nursing Facility Care Coinsurance			✓	✓	✓	✓	50%	75%	✓	✓
Medicare Part A Deductible		✓	✓	✓	✓	✓	50%	75%	50%	✓
Medicare Part B Deductible			✓		✓					
Medicare Part B Excess Charges					✓	✓				
Foreign Travel Emergency (Up to Plan Limits)			✓	✓	✓	✓			✓	✓
							Out-of-Pocket Limit**			
							$4,660	$2,330		

*Plan F also offers a high-deductible plan. If you choose this option, this means you must pay for Medicare-covered costs up to the deductible amount of $2,070 in 2012 before your Medigap plan pays anything.

** After you meet your out-of-pocket yearly limit and your yearly Part B deductible ($140 in 2012), the Medigap plan pays 100% of covered services for the rest of the calendar year.

***Plan N pays 100% of the Part B coinsurance, except for a copayment of up to $20 for some office visits and up to a $50 copayment for emergency room visits that don't result in an inpatient admission.

What Medigap Policies Don't Cover

Generally, Medigap policies don't cover long-term care (like care in a nursing home), vision or dental care, hearing aids, eyeglasses, or private-duty nursing.

Types of Coverage That Are NOT Medigap Policies

- Medicare Advantage Plans (Part C), like an HMO, PPO, or Private Fee-for-Service Plan
- Medicare Prescription Drug Plans (Part D)
- Medicaid
- Employer or union plans, including the Federal Employees Health Benefits Program (FEHBP)
- TRICARE
- Veterans' benefits
- Long-term care insurance policies
- Indian Health Service, Tribal, and Urban Indian Health plans

What Types of Medigap Policies Can Insurance Companies Sell?

In most cases, Medigap insurance companies can sell you only a "standardized" Medigap policy. All Medigap policies must have specific benefits so you can compare them easily.

Insurance companies that sell Medigap policies don't have to offer every Medigap plan. However, they must offer Medigap Plan A if they offer any Medigap policy. If they offer any plan in addition to Plan A, they must also offer Plan C or Plan F. Each insurance company decides which Medigap policies it wants to sell, although state laws might affect which ones they offer.

In some cases, an insurance company must sell you a Medigap policy, even if you have health problems. Listed below are certain times that you're guaranteed the right to buy a Medigap policy:

- When you're in your Medigap open enrollment period.
- If you have a guaranteed issue right.

You may also buy a Medigap policy at other times, but the insurance company can deny you a Medigap policy based on your health. Also, in some cases it may be illegal for the insurance company to sell you a Medigap policy (such as if you already have Medicaid or a Medicare Advantage Plan).

What Do I Need to Know if I Want to Buy a Medigap Policy?

- You must have Medicare Part A and Part B to buy a Medigap policy.
- If you have a Medicare Advantage Plan but are planning to return to Original Medicare, you can apply for a Medigap policy before your coverage ends. The Medigap insurer can sell it to you as long as you're leaving the plan. Ask that the new policy start no later than when your Medicare Advantage Plan enrollment ends, so you will have continuous coverage.
- Plans E, H, I, and J are no longer for sale, but you can keep these plans if you already have one.
- You pay the private insurance company a monthly premium for your Medigap policy in addition to the monthly Part B premium that you pay to Medicare.
- A Medigap policy only covers one person. If you and your spouse both want Medigap coverage, **you each will have to buy separate Medigap policies**.
- You can buy a Medigap policy from any insurance company that's licensed in your state to sell one.
- If you want to buy a Medigap policy, see the Medigap Plans chart to review the benefit choices. Then, follow the "**Steps to Buying a Medigap Policy**" in Section 4.
- If you want to drop your Medigap policy, write your insurance company to cancel the policy and confirm it's cancelled. Your agent can't cancel the policy for you.
- Any standardized Medigap policy is guaranteed renewable even if you have health problems. This means the insurance company can't cancel your Medigap policy as long as you pay the premium.
- Cost is usually the only difference between Medigap policies with the same letter sold by different insurance companies.
- Although some Medigap policies sold in the past covered prescription drugs, Medigap policies sold after January 1, 2006, aren't allowed to include prescription drug coverage.

- If you want prescription drug coverage, you can join a Medicare Prescription Drug Plan (Part D) offered by private companies approved by Medicare.

To learn about Medicare prescription drug coverage, visit www.medicare.gov/publications to view the booklet "Your Guide to Medicare Prescription Drug Coverage," or call 1-800-MEDICARE (1-800-633-4227). TTY users should call 1-877-486-2048.

When Is the Best Time to Buy a Medigap Policy?

The best time to buy a Medigap policy is during your Medigap open enrollment period. This period lasts for 6 months and begins on the first day of the month in which you're both 65 or older and enrolled in Medicare Part B. Some states have additional open enrollment periods including those for people under 65. During this period, an insurance company can't use medical underwriting. This means the insurance company can't do any of the following because of your health problems:

- Refuse to sell you any Medigap policy it offers
- Charge you more for a Medigap policy than they charge someone with no health problems
- Make you wait for coverage to start (except as explained below)

While the insurance company can't make you wait for your coverage to start, it may be able to make you wait for coverage related to a pre-existing condition. A preexisting condition is a health problem you have before the date a new insurance policy starts. In some cases, the Medigap insurance company can refuse to cover your out-of-pocket costs for these pre-existing health problems for up to 6 months. This is called a "pre-existing condition waiting period." After 6 months, the Medigap policy will cover the pre-existing condition. Coverage for a pre-existing condition can only be excluded in a Medigap policy if the condition was treated or diagnosed within 6 months before the date the coverage starts under the Medigap policy. This is called the "look-back period." After the 6-month pre-existing waiting period, the Medigap policy will cover the condition that was excluded. Remember, for Medicare-covered services, Original Medicare will still cover the condition, even if the Medigap policy won't cover your out-of-pocket costs, but you're responsible for the coinsurance or copayment.

If you have a pre-existing condition and you buy a Medigap policy during your Medigap open enrollment period and you're replacing certain kinds of health coverage that count as "creditable coverage," it's possible to avoid or shorten waiting periods for pre-existing conditions. Prior creditable coverage is generally any other health coverage you recently had before applying for a Medigap policy. If you have had at least 6 months of continuous prior creditable coverage, the Medigap insurance company can't make you wait before it covers your pre-existing conditions.

There are many types of health care coverage that may count as creditable coverage for Medigap policies, but they will only count if you didn't have a break in coverage for more than 63 days.

Talk to your Medigap insurance company. It will be able to tell you if your previous coverage will count as creditable coverage for this purpose. You can also call your State Health Insurance Assistance Program.

If you buy a Medigap policy when you have a guaranteed issue right (also called "Medigap protection"), the insurance company can't use a pre-existing condition waiting period.

Note: If you're under 65 and have Medicare, generally because of a disability or ESRD, you might not be able to buy the Medigap policy you want, or any Medigap policy, until you turn 65. Federal law doesn't require insurance companies to sell Medigap policies to people under 65. However, some states require Medigap insurance companies to sell you a Medigap policy, even if you're under 65.

Why Is It Important to Buy a Medigap Policy When I'm First Eligible?

It's very important to understand your Medigap open enrollment period. Medigap insurance companies are generally allowed to use medical underwriting to decide whether to accept your application and how much to charge you for the Medigap policy. However, if you apply during your Medigap open enrollment period, you can buy any Medigap policy the company sells, even if you have health problems, for the same price as people with good health. If you apply for Medigap coverage **after** your open enrollment period, there is no guarantee that an insurance company will sell you a Medigap policy if you don't meet the medical underwriting requirements, **unless** you're eligible because of one of the limited situations listed in Section 3.

It's also important to understand that your Medigap rights may depend on when you choose to enroll in Medicare Part B. If you're 65 or older, your Medigap open enrollment period begins when you enroll in Part B **and** can't be changed or repeated. In most cases, it makes sense to enroll in Part B when you're first eligible, because you might otherwise have to pay a Part B late enrollment penalty.

However, if you have group health coverage through an employer or union, because either you or your spouse is currently working, you may want to wait to enroll in Part B.

This is because employer plans often provide coverage similar to Medigap, so you don't need a Medigap policy. When your employer coverage ends, you will get a chance to enroll in Part B without a late enrollment penalty which means your Medigap open enrollment period will start when you're ready to take advantage of it. If you enrolled in Part B while you still had the employer coverage, your Medigap open enrollment period would start, and unless you bought a Medigap policy before you needed it, you would miss your open enrollment period entirely. If you or your spouse is still working and you have coverage through an employer, contact your employer or union benefits administrator to find out how your insurance works with Medicare.

How Do Insurance Companies Set Prices for Medigap Policies?

Each insurance company decides how it will set the price, or premium, for its Medigap policies. It's important to ask how an insurance company prices its policies. The way they set the price affects how much you pay now and in the future. Medigap policies can be priced or "rated" in three ways:

1) Community-rated (also called "no-age-rated")
2) Issue-age-rated (also called "entry-age-rated")
3) Attained-age-rated

Each of these ways of pricing Medigap policies is described in the chart on the next page. The examples show how your age affects your premiums, and why it's important to look at how much the Medigap policy will cost you now and in the future.

The amounts in the examples aren't actual costs. Other factors such as geographical rating, medical underwriting, and discounts can also affect the amount of your premiums.

Type of pricing	How it's priced	What this pricing may mean for you	Examples
Community-rated (also called "no-age- rated")	Generally the same monthly premium is charged to everyone who has the Medigap policy, regardless of age.	Your premium isn't based on your age. Premiums may go up because of inflation and other factors but not because of your age.	Mr. Smith is 65. He buys a Medigap policy and pays a $165 monthly premium. Mrs. Perez is 72. She buys the same Medigap policy as Mr. Smith. She also pays a $165 monthly premium because, with this type of Medigap policy, everyone pays the same price regardless of age.
Issue-age- rated (also called "entry age-rated")	The premium is based on the age you are when you buy (are "issued") the Medigap policy.	Premiums are lower for people who buy at a younger age and won't change as you get older. Premiums may go up because of inflation and other factors but not because of your age.	Mr. Han is 65. He buys a Medigap policy and pays a $145 monthly premium. Mrs. Wright is 72. She buys the same Medigap policy as Mr. Han. Since she is older when she buys it, her monthly premium is $175.
Attained-age-rated	The premium is based on your current age (the age you have "attained"), so your premium goes up as you get older.	Premiums are low for younger buyers but go up as you get older. They may be the least expensive at first, but they can eventually become the most expensive. Premiums may also go up because of inflation and other factors.	Mrs. Anderson is 65. She buys a Medigap policy and pays a $120 monthly premium. • At 66, her premium goes up to $126. • At 67, her premium goes up to $132. • At 72, her premium goes up to $165. Mr. Dodd is 72. He buys the same Medigap policy as Mrs. Anderson. He pays a $165 monthly premium. His premium is higher than Mrs. Anderson's because it's based on his current age. Mr. Dodd's premium will go up each year. • At 73, his premium goes up to $171. • At 74, his premium goes up to $177.

Comparing Medigap Costs

As discussed on the previous pages, the cost of Medigap policies can vary widely. **There can be big differences in the premiums that different insurance companies charge for exactly the same coverage**. As you shop for a Medigap policy, be sure to compare the same type of Medigap policy, and consider the type of pricing used. For example, compare a Medigap Plan C from one insurance company with a Medigap Plan C from another insurance company. Although this guide **can't** give actual costs of Medigap policies, you can get this information by calling insurance companies or your State Health Insurance Assistance Program.

You can also find out which insurance companies sell Medigap policies in your area by visiting www.medicare.gov/medigap.

The cost of your Medigap policy may also depend on whether the insurance company does any of the following:

- Offers discounts (such as discounts for women, non-smokers, or people who are married; discounts for paying yearly; discounts for paying your premiums using electronic funds transfer; or discounts for multiple policies).
- Uses medical underwriting, or applies a different premium when you don't have a guaranteed issue right, or aren't in a Medigap open enrollment period.
- Sells Medicare SELECT policies that may require you to use certain providers. If you buy this type of Medigap policy, your premium may be less.
- Offers a "high-deductible option" for Medigap Plan F. If you buy Medigap Plan F with a high-deductible option, you must pay the first $2,070 (in 2012) of deductibles, copayments, and coinsurance not paid by Medicare before the Medigap policy pays anything. You must also pay a separate deductible ($250 per year) for foreign travel emergency services.
- If you bought your Medigap Plan J before January 1, 2006, and it still covers prescription drugs, you would also pay a separate deductible ($250 per year) for prescription drugs covered by the Medigap policy. And, if you have a Plan J with a high deductible option, you must pay a $2,070 deductible before the policy pays anything.

What is Medicare SELECT?

Medicare SELECT is a type of Medigap policy sold in some states that requires you to use hospitals and, in some cases, doctors within its network to be eligible for full insurance benefits (except in an emergency). Medicare SELECT can be any of the standardized Medigap Plans. These policies generally cost less than other Medigap policies. However, if you don't use a Medicare SELECT hospital or doctor for non-emergency services, you will have to pay some or all of what Medicare doesn't pay. Medicare will pay its share of approved charges no matter which hospital or doctor you choose.

How Does Medigap Help Pay Your Medicare Part B Bills?

In most Medigap policies, when you sign the Medigap insurance contract you agree to have the Medigap insurance company get your Medicare Part B claim information directly from Medicare, and then they pay the doctor directly. Some Medigap insurance companies also provide this service for Medicare Part A claims.

If your Medigap insurance company **doesn't** provide this service, ask your doctors if they "participate" in Medicare. This means that they "accept assignment" for all Medicare patients. If your doctor participates, the Medigap insurance company is required to pay the doctor directly if you request.

If you have any questions about Medigap claim filing, call 1-800-MEDICARE (1-800-633-4227). TTY users should call 1-877-486-2048.

Section 3. Your Right to Buy a Medigap Policy

What Are Guaranteed Issue Rights?

The best time to buy a Medigap policy is during your Medigap open enrollment period, when you have the right to buy any Medigap policy offered in your state.

However, even if you aren't in your Medigap open enrollment period, there are several situations in which you may still have a guaranteed right to buy a Medigap policy if you're 65 or older.

Guaranteed issue rights (also called "Medigap protections") are rights you have in certain situations when insurance companies must offer you certain Medigap policies. In these situations, an insurance company must do the following:

- Sell you a Medigap policy
- Cover all your pre-existing health conditions
- Can't charge you more for a Medigap policy regardless of past or present health problems

If you live in Massachusetts, Minnesota, or Wisconsin, you have guaranteed issue rights to buy a Medigap policy, but the Medigap policies are different.

When Do I Have Guaranteed Issue Rights?

In most cases, you have a guaranteed issue right when you have other health care coverage that changes in some way, such as when you lose the other health care coverage.

In other cases, you have a "trial right" to try a Medicare Advantage Plan and still buy a Medigap policy if you change your mind.

An insurance company can't refuse to sell you a Medigap policy in the following situations

You have a guaranteed issue right if...	You have the right to buy...	You can/must apply for a Medigap policy...
You're in a Medicare Advantage Plan, and your plan is leaving Medicare or stops giving care in your area, or you move out of the plan's service area.	Medigap Plan A, B, C, F, K, or L that's sold in your state by any insurance company. You only have this right if you switch to Original Medicare rather than join another Medicare Advantage Plan.	As early as 60 calendar days before the date your health care coverage will end, but no later than 63 calendar days after your health care coverage ends. Medigap coverage can't start until your Medicare Advantage Plan coverage ends.

(Continued)

You have Original Medicare and an employer group health plan (including retiree or COBRA coverage) or union coverage that pays after Medicare pays and that plan is ending. Note: In this situation, you may have additional rights under state law.	Medigap Plan A, B, C, F, K, or L that's sold in your state by any insurance company. If you have COBRA coverage, you can either buy a Medigap policy right away or wait until the COBRA coverage ends.	No later than 63 calendar days after the latest of these 3 dates: 1. Date the coverage ends 2. Date on the notice you get telling you that coverage is ending (if you get one) 3. Date on a claim denial, if this is the only way you know that your coverage ended
You have Original Medicare and a Medicare SELECT policy. You move out of the Medicare SELECT policy's service area. Call the Medicare SELECT insurer for more information about your options.	Medigap Plan A, B, C, F, K, or L that's sold by any insurance company in your state or the state you're moving to.	As early as 60 calendar days before the date your Medicare SELECT coverage will end, but no later than 63 calendar days after your Medicare SELECT coverage ends.
(Trial Right) You joined a Medicare Advantage Plan or Programs of All-inclusive Care for the Elderly (PACE) when you were first eligible for Medicare Part A at 65, and within the first year of joining, you decide you want to switch to Original Medicare.	Any Medigap policy that's sold in your state by any insurance company.	As early as 60 calendar days before the date your coverage will end, but no later than 63 calendar days after your coverage ends. **Note:** Your rights may last for an extra 12 months under certain circumstances.
(Trial Right) You dropped a Medigap policy to join a Medicare Advantage Plan (or to switch to a Medicare SELECT policy) for the first time, you have been in the plan less than a year, and you want to switch back.	The Medigap policy you had before you joined the Medicare Advantage Plan or Medicare SELECT policy, if the same insurance company you had before still sells it. If your former Medigap policy isn't available, you can buy Medigap Plan A, B, C, F, K, orL that's sold in your state by any insurance company.	As early as 60 calendar days before the date your coverage will end, but no later than 63 calendar days after your coverage ends. Note: Your rights may last for an extra 12 months under certain circumstances.
Your Medigap insurance company goes bankrupt and you lose your coverage, or your Medigap policy coverage otherwise ends through no fault of your own.	Medigap Plan A, B, C, F, K, orL that's sold in your state by any insurance company.	No later than 63 calendar days from the date your coverage ends.
You leave a Medicare Advantage Plan or drop a Medigap policy because the company hasn't followed the rules, or it misled you.	Medigap Plan A, B, C, F, K, orL that's sold in your state by any insurance company.	No later than 63 calendar days from the date your coverage ends.

Can I Buy a Medigap Policy if I Lose My Health Care Coverage?

Because you may have a guaranteed issue right to buy a Medigap policy, make sure you keep the following:

- A copy of any letters, notices, emails, and/or claim denials that have your name on them as proof of your coverage being terminated
- The postmarked envelope these papers come in as proof of when it was mailed

You may need to send a copy of some or all of these papers with your Medigap application to prove you have a guaranteed issue right.

If you have a Medicare Advantage Plan but you're planning to return to Original Medicare, you can apply for a Medigap policy before your coverage ends. The Medigap insurer can sell it to you as long as you're leaving the plan. Ask that the new policy take effect no later than when your Medicare Advantage enrollment ends, so you will have continuous coverage.

For More Information

If you have any questions or want to learn about any additional Medigap rights in your state, you can do the following:

- Call your State Health Insurance Assistance Program to make sure that you qualify for these guaranteed issue rights.
- Call your State Insurance Department if you're denied Medigap coverage in any of these situations.

Important: The guaranteed issue rights in this section are from Federal law. These rights are for both Medigap and Medicare SELECT policies. Many states provide additional Medigap rights.

There may be times when more than one of the situations in the chart applies to you. When this happens, you can choose the guaranteed issue right that gives you the best choice. Some of the situations listed include loss of coverage under Programs of All-inclusive Care for the Elderly (PACE). PACE combines medical, social, and long-term care services, and prescription drug coverage for frail people. To be eligible for PACE, you must meet certain conditions. PACE may be available in states that have chosen it as an optional Medicaid benefit. If you have Medicaid, an insurance company can sell you a Medigap policy only in certain situations.

For more information about PACE, call 1-800-MEDICARE (1-800-633-4227). TTY users should call 1-877-486-2048.

Section 4. Steps to Buying a Medigap Policy

Step-by-Step Guide to Buying a Medigap Policy

Buying a **Medigap policy** is an important decision. Only you can decide if a Medigap policy is the way for you to supplement Original Medicare coverage and which Medigap policy to choose. Shop carefully. Compare available Medigap policies to see which one meets your needs. As you shop for a Medigap policy, keep in mind that different insurance companies may charge different amounts for exactly the same Medigap policy, and not all insurance companies offer all of the Medigap policies. Below is a step-by-step guide to help you buy a Medigap policy. If you live in Massachusetts, Minnesota, or Wisconsin, see Section 7.

STEP 1: Decide which benefits you want, then decide which of the Medigap Plans A through N meet your needs.

STEP 2: Find out which insurance companies sell Medigap policies in your state.

STEP 3: Call the insurance companies that sell the Medigap policies you're interested in and compare costs.

STEP 4: Buy the Medigap policy.

Step 1: Decide Which Benefits You Want, Then Decide Which of the Medigap Plans Meets Your Needs

You should think about your current and future health care needs when deciding which benefits you want because you might not be able to switch Medigap policies later. Decide which benefits you need, and select the Medigap policy that will work best for you.

Step 2: Find out Which Insurance Companies Sell Medigap Policies in Your State

To find out which insurance companies sell Medigap policies in your state, you can do any of the following:

- Call your State Health Insurance Assistance Program. Ask if they have a "Medigap rate comparison shopping guide" for your state. This guide usually lists companies that sell Medigap policies in your state and their costs.
- Call your State Insurance Department.
- Visit www.medicare.gov/medigap.

This Web site will help you find information on all your health plan options, including the Medigap policies in your area. You can also get information on the following:

- How to contact the insurance companies that sell Medigap policies in your state
- What each Medigap policy covers
- How insurance companies decide what to charge you for a Medigap policy premium

If you don't have a computer, your local library or senior center may be able to help you look at this information. You can also call 1-800-MEDICARE (1-800-633-4227). A customer service representative will help you get information on all your health plan options including the Medigap policies in your area. TTY users should call 1-877-486-2048. Since costs can vary between companies, you should plan to call more than one insurance company that sells Medigap policies in your state. Before you call, check the companies to be sure they're honest and reliable by using one of the resources listed below.

- Call your State Insurance Department. Ask if they keep a record of complaints against insurance companies that can be shared with you. When deciding which Medigap policy is right for you, consider any complaints against the insurance company.
- Call your State Health Insurance Assistance Program. These programs can give you free help with choosing a Medigap policy.

- Go to your local public library for help with the following:
  - Getting information on an insurance company's financial strength from independent rating services such as The Street.com Ratings, A.M. Best, and Standard & Poor's.
  - Looking at information about the insurance company online.
- Talk to someone you trust, like a family member, your insurance agent, or a friend who has a Medigap policy from the same Medigap insurance company.

Step 3: Call the Insurance Companies That Sell the Medigap Policies You're Interested in and Compare Costs

Before you call any insurance companies, figure out if you're in your Medigap open enrollment period or if you have a guaranteed issue right. Read pages 14–15 and 22–23 carefully. If you have questions, call your State Health Insurance Assistance Program. The chart below can help you keep track of the information you get.

Ask each insurance company…	Company 1	Company 2
"Are you licensed in ___?" (Say the name of your state.) Note: If the answer is NO, stop right here, and try another company.		
"Do you sell Medigap Plan ___?" (Say the letter of the Medigap Plan you're interested in.) Note: Insurance companies usually offer some, but not all, Medigap policies. Make sure the company sells the plan you want. Also, if you're interested in a Medicare SELECT or high-deductible Medigap policy, say so.		
"Do you use medical underwriting for this Medigap policy?" Note: If the answer is NO, go to step 4. If the answer is YES, but you know you're in your Medigap open enrollment period or have a guaranteed issue right to buy that Medigap policy, go to step 4. Otherwise, you can ask, "Can you tell me whether I am likely to qualify for the Medigap policy?"		
"Do you have a waiting period for pre-existing conditions?" Note: If the answer is YES, ask how long the waiting period is and write it in the box.		
"Do you price this Medigap policy by using community-rating, issue-age-rating, or attained-age-rating?" Note: Circle the one that applies for that insurance company.	Community Issue-age Attained-age	Community Issue-age Attained-age

"I am ___ years old. What would my premium be under this Medigap policy?" Note: If it's attained-age, ask, "How frequently does the premium increase due to my age?"		
"Has the premium for this Medigap policy increased in the last 3 years due to inflation or other reasons?" Note: If the answer is YES, ask how much it has increased, and write it in the box.		
"Do you offer any discounts or additional (innovative) benefits?"		
"Is there any extra charge to process my claims automatically?"		

Watch out for Illegal Insurance Practices

It's illegal for anyone to do the following:

- Pressure you into buying a Medigap policy, or lie to or mislead you to switch from one company or policy to another.
- Sell you a second Medigap policy when they know that you already have one, unless you tell the insurance company in writing that you plan to cancel your existing Medigap policy.
- Sell you a Medigap policy if they know you have Medicaid, except in certain situations.
- Sell you a Medigap policy if they know you're in a Medicare Advantage Plan (like an HMO, PPO, or Private Fee-for-Service Plan) unless your coverage under the Medicare Advantage Plan will end before the effective date of the Medigap policy.
- Claim that a Medigap policy is part of the Medicare Program or any other Federal program. Medigap is private health insurance.
- Claim that a Medicare Advantage Plan is a Medigap policy.
- Sell you a Medigap policy that can't legally be sold in your state. Check with your State Insurance Department to make sure that the Medigap policy you're interested in can be sold in your state.
- Misuse the names, letters, or symbols of the U.S. Department of Health & Human Services (HHS), Social Security Administration (SSA), Centers for Medicare & Medicaid Services (CMS), or any of their various programs like Medicare. (For example, they can't suggest the Medigap policy has been approved or recommended by the Federal government.)

- Claim to be a Medicare representative if they work for a Medigap insurance company.
- Sell you a Medicare Advantage Plan when you say you want to stay in Original Medicare and buy a Medigap policy. A Medicare Advantage Plan isn't the same as Original Medicare. If you enroll in a Medicare Advantage Plan, you can't use a Medigap policy.

If you believe that a Federal law has been broken, call the Inspector General's hotline at 1-800-HHS-TIPS (1-800-447-8477). TTY users should call 1-800-377-4950. Your State Insurance Department can help you with other insurance-related problems.

Step 4: Buy the Medigap Policy

Once you decide on the insurance company and the Medigap policy you want, you should apply. The insurance company must give you a clearly worded summary of your Medigap policy. Read it carefully. If you don't understand it, ask questions. Remember the following when you buy your Medigap policy:

- Filling out your application. Fill out the application carefully and completely, including medical questions. The answers you give will determine your eligibility for open enrollment or guaranteed issue rights. If the insurance agent fills out the application, make sure it's correct. If you buy a Medigap policy during your Medigap open enrollment period or provide evidence that you're entitled to a guaranteed issue right, the insurance company can't use any medical answers you give to deny you a Medigap policy or change the price. The insurance company can't ask you any questions about your family history or require you to take a genetic test.
- Paying for your Medigap policy. It's best to pay for your Medigap policy by check, money order, or bank draft. Make it payable to the insurance company, not the agent. If buying from an agent, get a receipt with the insurance company's name, address, and phone number for your records. Some companies may offer electronic funds transfer.
- Starting your Medigap policy. Ask for your Medigap policy to become effective when you want coverage to start. Generally,

Medigap policies begin the first of the month after you apply. If, for any reason, the insurance company won't give you the effective date for the month you want, call your State Insurance Department.

Note: If you already have a Medigap policy, ask for your new Medigap policy to become effective when your old Medigap policy coverage ends.

- **Getting your Medigap policy.** If you don't get your Medigap policy in 30 days, call your insurance company. If you don't get your Medigap policy in 60 days, call your State Insurance Department.

If you already have a Medigap policy, it's illegal for an insurance company to sell you a second policy unless you tell them in writing that you will cancel the first Medigap policy. However, don't cancel your old Medigap policy until the new one is in place, and you decide to keep it. Once you get the new Medigap policy, you have 30 days to decide if you want to keep the new policy. This is called your "free look" period. The 30-day free look period begins on the day you get your Medigap policy. You will need to pay both premiums for one month.

Section 5. For People Who Already Have a Medigap Policy

You should read this section if any of these situations apply to you:

- You're thinking about switching to a different Medigap policy.
- You're losing your Medigap coverage.
- You have a Medigap policy with Medicare prescription drug coverage.

Switching Medigap Policies

If you're satisfied with your current Medigap policy's cost, coverage, and customer service, you don't need to do anything. If you're thinking about switching to a new Medigap policy, see below to answer some common questions about switching Medigap policies.

Can I Switch to a Different Medigap Policy?

In most cases, you won't have a right under Federal law to switch Medigap policies, unless you're within your 6-month Medigap open enrollment period or are eligible under a specific circumstance for guaranteed issue rights. But, if your state has more generous requirements, or the insurance company is willing to sell you a Medigap policy, make sure you compare benefits and premiums before switching. If you bought your Medigap policy before 2010, it may offer coverage that isn't available in a newer Medigap policy. On the other hand, Medigap policies bought before 1992 might not be guaranteed renewable and might have bigger premium increases than newer, standardized Medigap policies currently being sold.

If you decide to switch, don't cancel your first Medigap policy until you have decided to keep the second Medigap policy. On the application for the new Medigap policy, you will have to promise that you will cancel your first Medigap policy. You have 30 days to decide if you want to keep the new Medigap policy. This is called your "free look period." The 30-day free look period starts when you get your new Medigap policy. You will need to pay both premiums for one month.

Do I Have to Switch Medigap Policies if I Have an Older Medigap Policy?

No. But if you buy a new Medigap policy, you have to give up your old policy (except for your 30-day "free look period,"). Once you cancel the policy, you can't get it back, and it can no longer be sold because it isn't a standardized policy.

Do I Have to Wait a Certain Length of Time after I Buy My First Medigap Policy before I Can Switch to a Different Medigap Policy?

No. You should be aware that if you've had your old Medigap policy for less than 6 months, the Medigap insurance company may be able to make you wait up to 6 months for coverage of a pre-existing condition. However, if your old Medigap policy had the same benefits, and you had it for 6 months or more, the new insurance company can't exclude your pre-existing condition. If you've had your Medigap policy less than 6 months, the number of months you've had your current Medigap policy must be subtracted from the time you must wait before your new Medigap policy covers your pre-existing condition.

If the new Medigap policy has a benefit that isn't in your current Medigap policy, you may still have to wait up to 6 months before that benefit will be covered, regardless of how long you've had your current Medigap policy.

If you've had your current Medigap policy longer than 6 months and want to replace it with a new one with the same benefits and the insurance company agrees to issue the new policy, they can't write pre-existing conditions, waiting periods, elimination periods, or probationary periods into the replacement policy.

Why Would I Want to Switch to a Different Medigap Policy?

Some reasons for switching may include the following:

- You're paying for benefits you don't need.
- You need more benefits than you needed before.
- Your current Medigap policy has the right benefits, but you want to change your insurance company.
- Your current Medigap policy has the right benefits, but you want to find a policy that's less expensive.

It's important to compare the benefits in your current Medigap policy to the benefits listed in the Medigap Plans chart. To help you compare benefits and decide which Medigap policy you want, follow the "**Steps to Buying a Medigap Policy**" in Section 4. If you decide to change insurance companies, you can call the new insurance company and arrange to apply for your new Medigap policy. If your application is accepted, call your current insurance company, and ask to have your coverage end. The insurance company can tell you how to submit a request to end your coverage.

You should have your old Medigap policy coverage end **after** you have the new Medigap policy for 30 days. Remember, this is your 30-day free look period. You will need to pay both premiums for one month.

Can I Keep My Current Medigap Policy (or Medicare SELECT Policy) or Switch to a Different Medigap Policy if I Move out-of-State?

You can keep your current Medigap policy regardless of where you live as long as you still have Original Medicare. If you want to switch to a different Medigap policy, you will have to check with your current or the new insurance company to see if they will offer you a different Medigap policy.

You may have to pay more for your new Medigap policy and answer some medical questions if you're buying a Medigap policy outside of your Medigap open enrollment period.

If you have a Medicare SELECT policy and you move out of the policy's area, you have the following choices:

- Buy a standardized Medigap policy from your current Medigap policy insurance company that offers the same or fewer benefits than your current Medicare SELECT policy. If you've had your Medicare SELECT policy for more than 6 months, you won't have to answer any medical questions.
- You have a guaranteed issue right to buy any Medigap Plan A, B, C, F, K, or L that's sold in most states by any insurance company.

What Happens to My Medigap Policy if I Join a Medicare Advantage Plan?

Medigap policies can't work with Medicare Advantage Plans. If you decide to keep your Medigap policy, you will have to pay your Medigap policy premium, but the Medigap policy can't pay any deductibles, copayments, coinsurance, or premiums under a Medicare Advantage Plan. So, if you want to join a Medicare Advantage Plan, you may want to drop your Medigap policy. Contact your Medigap insurance company to find out how to disenroll.

However, if you leave the Medicare Advantage Plan you might not be able to get the same Medigap policy back, or in some cases, any Medigap policy unless you have a "trial right." Your rights to buy a Medigap policy may vary by state. You always have a legal right to keep the Medigap policy after you join a Medicare Advantage Plan. However, because you have a Medicare Advantage Plan, the Medigap policy would no longer provide benefits that supplement Medicare.

Losing Medigap Coverage

Can My Medigap Insurance Company Drop Me?

If you bought your Medigap policy **after 1992**, in most cases the Medigap insurance company can't drop you because the Medigap policy is guaranteed renewable. This means your insurance company can't drop you unless one of the following happens:

- You stop paying your premium.
- You weren't truthful on the Medigap policy application.
- The insurance company becomes bankrupt or insolvent.

However, if you bought your Medigap policy **before 1992**, it might not be guaranteed renewable. This means the Medigap insurance company can refuse to renew the Medigap policy, as long as it gets the state's approval to cancel your Medigap policy. However, if this does happen, you have the right to buy another Medigap policy. See the guaranteed issue right.

Medigap Policies and Medicare Prescription Drug Coverage

If you bought a Medigap policy **before** January 1, 2006, and it has coverage for prescription drugs, see below. Medicare offers prescription drug coverage (Part D) for everyone with Medicare. If you have a Medigap policy with prescription drug coverage, that means you chose not to join a Medicare Prescription Drug Plan when you were first eligible. However, you can still join a Medicare Prescription Drug Plan. Your situation may have changed in ways that make a Medicare Prescription Drug Plan fit your needs better than the prescription drug coverage in your Medigap policy. It's a good idea to review your coverage each fall, because you can join a Medicare Prescription Drug Plan between October 15–December 7. Your new coverage will begin on January 1.

Why Would I Change My Mind and Join a Medicare Prescription Drug Plan?

In a Medicare Prescription Drug Plan, you may have to pay a monthly premium, but Medicare pays a large part of the cost. There's no maximum yearly amount as with Medigap prescription drug benefits in old Plans H, I, and J (these plans are no longer sold). However, a Medicare Prescription Drug Plan might only cover certain prescription drugs (on its "formulary" or "drug list"). It's important that you check whether your current prescription drugs are on the Medicare Prescription Drug Plan's list of covered prescription drugs before you join. If your Medigap premium or your prescription drug needs were very low when you had your first chance to join a Medicare Prescription Drug Plan, your Medigap prescription drug coverage may have met your needs. However, if your Medigap premium or the amount of prescription drugs you use has increased recently, a Medicare Prescription Drug Plan might now be a better choice for you.

Will I Have to Pay a Late Enrollment Penalty if I Join a Medicare Prescription Drug Plan Now?

This will depend on whether your Medigap policy includes "creditable prescription drug coverage." This means that the Medigap policy's drug coverage pays, on average, at least as much as Medicare's standard prescription drug coverage.

If it **isn't** creditable coverage, and you join a Medicare Prescription Drug Plan now, you will probably pay a higher premium (a penalty added to your monthly premium) than if you had joined when you were first eligible. You should also consider that your prescription drug needs could increase as you get older. Each month that you wait to join a Medicare Prescription Drug Plan will make your late enrollment penalty higher.

Your Medigap carrier must send you a notice each year telling you if the prescription drug coverage in your Medigap policy is creditable. You should keep these notices in case you decide later to join a Medicare Prescription Drug Plan.

If your Medigap policy includes creditable coverage and you decide to join a Medicare Prescription Drug Plan, you won't have to pay a late enrollment penalty as long as you don't drop your Medigap policy **before** you join the Medicare Prescription Drug Plan. You can only join a Medicare Prescription Drug Plan between October 15–December 7 unless you lose your Medigap policy (for example, if it isn't guaranteed renewable, and your company cancels it). In that case, you may be able to join a Medicare Prescription Drug Plan at the time you lose your Medigap policy.

Can I Join a Medicare Prescription Drug Plan and Have a Medigap Policy with Prescription Drug Coverage?

No. If your Medigap policy covers prescription drugs, you must tell your Medigap insurance company if you join a Medicare Prescription Drug Plan so it can remove the prescription drug coverage from your Medigap policy and adjust your premium.

Once the drug coverage is removed, you can't get that coverage back even though you didn't change Medigap policies.

What if I Decide to Drop My Entire Medigap Policy (Not Just the Medigap Prescription Drug Coverage) and Join a Medicare Advantage Plan That Offers Prescription Drug Coverage?

You need to be careful about the timing because you can only join a Medicare Prescription Drug Plan or Medicare Advantage Plan during the open enrollment period between October 15–December 7. Your coverage will begin on January 1 as long as the plan gets your enrollment request by December 7.

Section 6. Medigap Policies for People with a Disability or ESRD

Information for People under 65

Medigap Policies for People under 65 and Eligible for Medicare Because of a Disability or End-Stage Renal Disease (ESRD)

You may have Medicare before 65 due to a disability or ESRD (permanent kidney failure requiring dialysis or a kidney transplant). If you're a person with Medicare under 65 and have a disability or ESRD, you might not be able to buy the Medigap policy you want, or any Medigap policy, until you turn 65. Federal law doesn't require insurance companies to sell Medigap policies to people under 65. However, some states require Medigap insurance companies to sell you a Medigap policy, even if you're under 65. These states are listed below.

Important: These are the minimum Federal standards. For your state requirements, call your State Health Insurance Assistance Program. At the time of printing this guide, the following states required insurance companies to offer at least one kind of Medigap policy to people with Medicare under 65:

- California*
- Colorado
- Connecticut
- Delaware**
- Florida
- Georgia
- Hawaii
- Illinois
- Kansas

- Louisiana
- Maine
- Maryland
- Massachusetts*
- Michigan
- Minnesota
- Mississippi
- Missouri
- New Hampshire
- New Jersey
- New York
- North Carolina
- Oklahoma
- Oregon
- Pennsylvania
- South Dakota
- Tennessee
- Texas
- Vermont*
- Wisconsin

* A Medigap policy isn't available to people with ESRD under 65.
** A Medigap policy is only available to people with ESRD.

Even if your state isn't on the list above, some insurance companies may voluntarily sell Medigap policies to people under 65, although they will probably cost you more than Medigap policies sold to people over 65, and they can use medical underwriting. Check with your state about what rights you might have under state law. Remember, if you're already enrolled in Medicare Part B, you will get a Medigap open enrollment period when you turn 65. You will probably have a wider choice of Medigap policies and be able to get a lower premium at that time. During the Medigap open enrollment period, insurance companies can't refuse to sell you any Medigap policy due to a disability or other health problem, or charge you a higher premium (based on health status) than they charge other people who are 65. Because Medicare (Part A and/or Part B) is creditable coverage, if you had Medicare for more than 6 months before you turned 65, you may not have a pre-existing condition waiting period. If you have questions, call your State Health Insurance Assistance Program.

Section 7. Medigap Coverage in Massachusetts, Minnesota, and Wisconsin

Massachusetts—Chart of standardized Medigap policies

Massachusetts Benefits

- Inpatient Hospital Care: Covers the Medicare Part A coinsurance plus coverage for 365 additional days after Medicare coverage ends
- Medical Costs: Covers the Medicare Part B coinsurance (generally 20% of the Medicare-approved amount)
- Blood: Covers the first 3 pints of blood each year
- Part A hospice coinsurance or copayment

The check marks in this chart mean the benefit is covered.

Medigap Benefits	Core Plan	Supplement 1 Plan
Basic Benefits	√	√
Medicare Part A: Inpatient Hospital Deductible		√
Medicare Part A: Skilled Nursing Facility Coinsurance		√
Medicare Part B: Deductible		√
Foreign Travel Emergency		√
Inpatient Days in Mental Health Hospitals	60 days per calendar year	120 days per benefit year
State-Mandated Benefits (Annual Pap tests and mammograms. Check your plan for other state-mandated benefits.)	√	√

For more information on these Medigap policies, visit www.medicare.gov/medigap, or call your State Insurance Department.

Minnesota—Chart of Standardized Medigap Policies

Minnesota Benefits

- **Inpatient Hospital Care:** Covers the Medicare Part A coinsurance
- **Medical Costs:** Covers the Medicare Part B coinsurance (generally 20% of the Medicare-approved amount)

- **Blood:** Covers the first 3 pints of blood each year
- Part A hospice and respite cost sharing
- Parts A and B home health services and supplies cost sharing

The check marks in this chart mean the benefit is covered.

<table>
<tr><th>Medigap Benefits</th><th>Basic Plan</th><th>Extended Basic Plan</th><th>Mandatory Riders</th></tr>
<tr><td>Basic Benefits</td><td>√</td><td>√</td><td rowspan="11">Insurance companies can offer four additional riders that can be added to a Basic Plan. You may choose any one or all of the following riders to design a Medigap policy that meets your needs:

• Medicare Part A: Inpatient Hospital Deductible
• Medicare Part B: Deductible
• Usual and Customary Fees
• Non-Medicare Preventive Care</td></tr>
<tr><td>Medicare Part A: Inpatient Hospital Deductible</td><td></td><td></td></tr>
<tr><td>Medicare Part A: Skilled Nursing Facility (SNF) Coinsurance</td><td>√ (Provides 100 days of SNF care)</td><td>√ (Provides 120 days of SNF care)</td></tr>
<tr><td>Medicare Part B: Deductible</td><td></td><td>√</td></tr>
<tr><td>Foreign Travel Emergency</td><td>80%</td><td>80%*</td></tr>
<tr><td>Outpatient Mental Health</td><td>50%</td><td>50%</td></tr>
<tr><td>Usual and Customary Fees</td><td></td><td>80%*</td></tr>
<tr><td>Medicare-covered Preventive Care</td><td>√</td><td>√</td></tr>
<tr><td>Physical Therapy</td><td>20%</td><td>20%</td></tr>
<tr><td>Coverage while in a Foreign Country</td><td></td><td>80%*</td></tr>
<tr><td>State-mandated Benefits (Diabetic equipment and supplies, routine cancer screening, reconstructive surgery, and immunizations)</td><td>√</td><td>√</td></tr>
</table>

*** Pays 100% after you spend $1,000 in out-of-pocket costs for a calendar year.**

Minnesota versions of Medigap Plans K, L, M, N, and high deductible F are available.

Important: The Basic and Extended Basic benefits are available when you enroll in Part B, regardless of age or health problems. If you return to work and drop Part B to elect your employer's health plan, you will get another 6-month Medigap open enrollment period after you retire from that employer when you can elect Part B again.

Wisconsin Benefits

- Inpatient Hospital Care: Covers the Part A coinsurance
- Medical Costs: Covers the Part B coinsurance (generally 20% of the Medicare-approved amount)
- Blood: Covers the first 3 pints of blood each year
- Part A Hospice coinsurance or copayment

The check marks in this chart mean the benefit is covered.

<table>
<tr><th>Medigap Benefits</th><th>Basic Plan</th><th>Optional Riders</th></tr>
<tr><td>Basic Benefits</td><td>√</td><td rowspan="5">Insurance companies are allowed to offer the following additional riders to a Medigap policy:
• Part A Deductible
• Additional Home Health Care (365 visits including those paid by Medicare)
• Part B Deductible
• Part B Excess Charges
• Foreign Travel Emergency
• 50% Part A Deductible
• Part B Copayment or Coinsurance</td></tr>
<tr><td>Medicare Part A: Skilled Nursing Facility Coinsurance</td><td>√</td></tr>
<tr><td>Inpatient Mental Health Coverage</td><td>175 days per lifetime in addition to Medicare's benefit</td></tr>
<tr><td>Home Health Care</td><td>40 visits in addition to those paid by Medicare</td></tr>
<tr><td>State Mandated Benefits</td><td>√</td></tr>
</table>

For more information on these Medigap policies, visit www.medicare.gov/medigap, or call your State Insurance Department.

Plans known as "50% and 25% Cost-sharing Plans" are available. These plans are similar to standardized Plans K (50%) and L (25%). A high deductible plan ($2,070 deductible for 2012) is also available.

Section 8. For More Information

Where to Get More Information

Below, you will find phone numbers for your State Health Insurance Assistance Program and State Insurance Department.

- Call your State Health Insurance Assistance Program for help with any of the following:
  - Buying a Medigap policy or long-term care insurance
  - Dealing with payment denials or appeals
  - Medicare rights and protections
  - Choosing a Medicare plan
  - Deciding whether to suspend your Medigap policy
  - Questions about Medicare bills
- Call your State Insurance Department if you have questions about the Medigap policies sold in your area or any insurance-related problems.

How to Get Help with Medicare and Medigap Questions

If you have questions about Medicare, Medigap, or need updated phone numbers for the contacts listed, you can do the following:

Visit www.medicare.gov:

- For Medigap policies in your area, visit www.medicare.gov/medigap
- For updated phone numbers, visit ww.medicare.gov/contacts.

Call 1-800-MEDICARE (1-800-633-4227):

- Customer service representatives are available 24 hours a day, 7 days a week. TTY users should call 1-877-486-2048. If you need help in a language other than English or Spanish, let the customer service representative know the language.

State Health Insurance Assistance Program and State Insurance Department

State	State Health Insurance Assistance Program	State Insurance Department
Alabama	1-800-243-5463	1-800-433-3966
Alaska	1-800-478-6065	1-800-467-8725
American Samoa	Not Available	1-684-633-4116
Arizona	1-800-432-4040	1-800-325-2548
Arkansas	1-800-224-6330	1-800-224-6330
California	1-800-434-0222	1-800-927-4357
Colorado	1-888-696-7213	1-800-930-3745

State	State Health Insurance Assistance Program	State Insurance Department
Connecticut	1-800-994-9422	1-800-203-3447
Delaware	1-800-336-9500	1-800-282-8611
Florida	1-800-963-5337	1-877-693-5236
Georgia	1-800-669-8387	1-800-656-2298
Guam	1-671-735-7388	1-671-635-1835
Hawaii	1-888-875-9229	1-808-586-2790
Idaho	1-800-247-4422	1-800-721-3272
Illinois	1-800-548-9034	1-866-445-5364
Indiana	1-800-452-4800	1-800-622-4461
Iowa	1-800-351-4664	1-877-955-1212
Kansas	1-800-860-5260	1-800-432-2484
Kentucky	1-877-293-7447	1-800-595-6053
Louisiana	1-800-259-5301	1-800-259-5300
Maine	1-877-353-3771	1-800-300-5000
Maryland	1-800-243-3425	1-800-492-6116
Massachusetts	1-800-243-4636	1-617-521-7794
Michigan	1-800-803-7174	1-877-999-6442
Minnesota	1-800-333-2433	1-800-657-3602
Mississippi	1-800-948-3090	1-800-562-2957
Missouri	1-800-390-3330	1-800-726-7390
Montana	1-800-551-3191	1-800-332-6148
Nebraska	1-800-234-7119	1-800-234-7119
Nevada	1-800-307-4444	1-800-992-0900
New Hampshire	1-866-634-9412	1-800-852-3416
New Jersey	1-800-792-8820	1-800-446-7467
New Mexico	1-800-432-2080	1-800-947-4722
New York	1-800-701-0501	1-800-342-3736
North Carolina	1-800-443-9354	1-800-546-5664
North Dakota	1-800-247-0560	1-800-247-0560
Northern Mariana Islands	Not Available	1-670-664-3064
Ohio	1-800-686-1578	1-800-686-1526
Oklahoma	1-800-763-2828	1-800-522-0071
Oregon	1-800-722-4134	1-888-877-4894
Pennsylvania	1-800-783-7067	1-877-881-6388
Puerto Rico	1-877-725-4300	1-888-722-8686
Rhode Island	1-401-462-0530	1-401-462-9520
South Carolina	1-800-868-9095	1-803-737-6160
South Dakota	1-877-331-4834	1-605-773-3563
Tennessee	1-877-801-0044	1-800-342-4029
Texas	1-800-252-9240	1-800-252-3439
Utah	1-877-424-4640	1-800-439-3805
Vermont	1-800-642-5119	1-800-631-7788
Virgin Islands	1-340-772-7368 1-340-714-4354 (St.Thomas)	1-340-774-7166
Virginia	1-800-552-3402	1-877-310-6560
Washington	1-800-562-6900	1-800-562-6900

(Continued)

State	State Health Insurance Assistance Program	State Insurance Department
Washington D.C.	1-202-994-6272	1-202-727-8000
West Virginia	1-877-987-4463	1-888-879-9842
Wisconsin	1-800-242-1060	1-800-236-8517
Wyoming	1-800-856-4398	1-800-438-5768

Section 9. Definitions

Assignment—An agreement by your doctor or other supplier to be paid directly by Medicare, to accept the payment amount Medicare approves for the service, and not to bill you for any more than the Medicare deductible and coinsurance.

Coinsurance—An amount you may be required to pay as your share of the costs for services after you pay any deductibles. Coinsurance is usually a percentage (for example, 20%).

Copayment—An amount you may be required to pay as your share of the cost for a medical service or supply, like a doctor's visit, hospital outpatient visit, or a prescription. A copayment is usually a set amount, rather than a percentage. For example, you might pay $10 or $20 for a doctor's visit or prescription.

Deductible—The amount you must pay for health care or prescriptions, before Original Medicare, your prescription drug plan, or your other insurance begins to pay.

Excess Charge—If you have Original Medicare, and the amount a doctor or other health care provider is legally permitted to charge is higher than the Medicare-approved amount, the difference is called the excess charge.

Guaranteed Issue Rights (also called "Medigap Protections")—Rights you have in certain situations when insurance companies are required by law to sell or offer you a Medigap policy. In these situations, an insurance company can't deny you a Medigap policy, or place conditions on a Medigap policy, such as exclusions for pre-existing conditions, and can't charge you more for a Medigap policy because of a past or present health problem.

Guaranteed Renewable Policy—An insurance policy can't be terminated by the insurance company unless you make untrue statements to the insurance company, commit fraud, or don't pay your premiums. All Medigap policies issued since 1992 are guaranteed renewable.

Medicaid—A joint Federal and state program that helps with medical costs for some people with limited income and resources. Medicaid programs vary from state to state, but most health care costs are covered if you qualify for both Medicare and Medicaid.

Medical Underwriting—The process that an insurance company uses to decide, based on your medical history, whether or not to take your application for insurance, whether or not to add a waiting period for pre-existing conditions (if your state law allows it), and how much to charge you for that insurance.

Medicare Advantage Plan (Part C)—A type of Medicare health plan offered by a private company that contracts with Medicare to provide you with all your Medicare Part A and Part B benefits. Medicare Advantage Plans include Health Maintenance Organizations, Preferred Provider Organizations, Private Fee-for-Service Plans, Special Needs Plans, and Medicare Medical Savings Account Plans. If you are enrolled in a Medicare Advantage Plan, Medicare services are covered through the plan and aren't paid for under Original Medicare. Most Medicare Advantage Plans offer prescription drug coverage.

Medicare-approved Amount—In Original Medicare, this is the amount a doctor or supplier that accepts assignment can be paid. It may be less than the actual amount a doctor or supplier charges. Medicare pays part of this amount and you are responsible for the difference.

Medicare Prescription Drug Plan (Part D)— A stand-alone drug plan that adds prescription drug coverage to Original Medicare, some Medicare Cost Plans, some Medicare PrivateFee-for-Service Plans, and Medicare Medical Savings Account Plans. If you have a Medigap policy without prescription drug coverage, you can also add a Medicare Prescription Drug Plan. These plans are offered by insurance companies and other private companies approved by Medicare. Medicare Advantage Plans may also offer prescription drug coverage that follows the same rules as Medicare Prescription Drug Plans.

Medicare SELECT—A type of Medigap policy that may require you to use hospitals and, in some cases, doctors within its network to be eligible for full benefits.

Open Enrollment Period (Medigap)—A one-time-only, 6-month period when Federal law allows you to buy any Medigap policy you want that is sold in your state. It starts in the first month that you're covered under Medicare Part B, **and** you're 65 or older. During this period, you can't be denied a Medigap policy or charged more due to past or present health problems. Some states may have additional open enrollment rights under state law.

Original Medicare—Original Medicare is fee-for-service coverage under which the government pays your health care providers directly for your Part A and/or Part B benefits.

Pre-existing Condition—A health problem you had before the date that a new insurance policy starts.

Premium—The periodic payment to Medicare, an insurance company, or a health care plan for health care or prescription drug coverage.

State Health Insurance Assistance Program (SHIP)—A state program that gets money from the Federal government to give free local health insurance counseling to people with Medicare.

State Insurance Department—A state agency that regulates insurance and can provide information about Medigap policies and other private health insurance.

Section 10. List of Topics

An alphabetical list of what's in this guide

Important Information about This Guide

The information, phone numbers, and web addresses in this guide were correct at the time of printing. Changes may occur after printing. To get the most up-to-date information and Medicare phone numbers, visit www.medicare.gov, or call 1-800-MEDICARE (1-800-633-4227). TTY users should call 1-877-486-2048.

The "2012 Choosing a Medigap Policy: A Guide to Health Insurance for People with Medicare" isn't a legal document. Official Medicare Program legal guidance is contained in the relevant statutes, regulations, and rulings.

In: Medigap
Editor: Johny P. Hughes
ISBN: 978-1-62417-279-3

Chapter 3

Medicare Primer*

Patricia A. Davis, Cliff Binder, Jim Hahn, Paulette C. Morgan, Janemarie Mulvey, Scott R. Talaga and Sibyl Tilson

Summary

Medicare is a federal insurance program that pays for covered health care services of qualified beneficiaries. It was established in 1965 under Title XVIII of the Social Security Act as a federal entitlement program to provide health insurance to individuals 65 and older, and has been expanded over the years to include permanently disabled individuals under 65. Medicare, which consists of four parts (A-D), covers hospitalizations, physician services, prescription drugs, skilled nursing facility care, home health visits, and hospice care, among other services.

Generally, individuals are eligible for Medicare if they or their spouse worked for at least 40 quarters in Medicare-covered employment, are 65 years old, and are a citizen or permanent resident of the United States. Individuals may also qualify for coverage if they are a younger person with a permanent disability, have End-Stage Renal disease (permanent kidney failure requiring dialysis or transplant), or have amyotrophic lateral sclerosis (ALS, Lou Gehrig's disease). In addition, individuals with one or more specified lung diseases or types of cancer

* This is an edited, reformatted and augmented version of Congressional Research Service, Publication No. R40425, dated April 24, 2012.

who lived for six months during a specified period prior to diagnosis in an area subject to a public health emergency declaration by the Environmental Protection Agency (EPA) as of June 17, 2009, are also deemed entitled to benefits under Part A and eligible to enroll in Part B.

In FY2012, the program will cover approximately 50 million persons (41 million aged and 9 million disabled) at a total cost of about $576 billion, accounting for approximately 3.7% of GDP. Medicare is an entitlement program, which means that it is required to pay for covered services provided to eligible persons so long as specific criteria are met.

Since 1965, the Medicare program has undergone considerable change. During the 111th Congress, the Patient Protection and Affordable Care Act (ACA; P.L. 111-148) and the Health Care and Education Affordability Reconciliation Act of 2010 (the Reconciliation Act, or HCERA; P.L. 111-152) were signed into law. They made numerous changes to the Medicare program that modify provider reimbursements, provide incentives to increase the quality and efficiency of care, and enhance certain Medicare benefits.

However, in the absence of congressional action, the Medicare program will be unsustainable in the long run. The Hospital Insurance (Part A) trust fund has been estimated to become insolvent in 2024. And although the Supplementary Medical Insurance (Parts B and D) trust fund is financed in large part through federal general revenues and cannot become insolvent, Medicare spending growth will put increasing strains on Congress's competing priorities.

The 112th Congress may continue to debate the recent changes to Medicare and may also consider additional legislative action ranging from technical corrections to broader structural changes. Additionally, Congress may consider legislative action to address the 2013-2021 automatic Medicare spending reductions under the Budget Control Act of 2011 (BCA; P.L. 112-25).

Introduction

Medicare is a federal insurance program that pays for covered health care services of qualified beneficiaries. It was established in 1965 under Title XVIII of the Social Security Act as a federal entitlement program to provide health insurance to individuals 65 and older, and has been expanded over the years to include permanently disabled individuals under 65. Medicare consists of four distinct parts:

- Part A (Hospital Insurance, or HI) covers inpatient hospital services, skilled nursing care, and home health and hospice care. The HI trust fund is mainly funded by a dedicated payroll tax of 2.9% of earnings, shared equally between employers and workers.

- Part B (Supplementary Medical Insurance, or SMI) covers physician services, outpatient services, and some home health and preventive services. The SMI trust fund is funded through beneficiary premiums (set at 25% of estimated program costs for the aged) and general revenues (the remaining amount, approximately 75%).
- Part C (Medicare Advantage, or MA) is a private plan option for beneficiaries that covers all Part A and B services, except hospice. Individuals choosing to enroll in Part C must also enroll in Part B. Part C is funded through the HI and SMI trust funds.
- Part D covers prescription drug benefits. Funding is included in the SMI trust fund and is financed through beneficiary premiums, general revenues, and state transfer payments.

Medicare serves approximately one in seven Americans and virtually all of the population aged 65 and over. In 2012, the program will cover an estimated 50 million persons (41 million aged and 9 million disabled). The Congressional Budget Office (CBO) estimates that total Medicare spending in 2012 will be about $575.7 billion, accounting for approximately 3.7% of GDP. In 2012, spending on benefits will be approximately $555.9 billion. Almost a third of Medicare benefit spending is for hospital services (see **Figure 1**). CBO also estimates that federal Medicare spending (after deduction of beneficiary premiums and other offsetting receipts) will be about $491.9 billion in 2012, accounting for about 13.6% of total federal spending. Medicare is an entitlement program, which means that it is required to pay for all covered services provided to eligible persons, so long as specific criteria are met. Spending under the program (except for a portion of administrative costs) is considered mandatory spending and is not subject to the appropriations process.

Medicare is expected to continue to be a high-priority issue in the second session of the 112th Congress. The program has a significant impact on the lives of millions of Americans and on the economy in general through its coverage of important health care benefits for the aged and disabled, the payment of premiums and other cost-sharing by those beneficiaries, and its payments to providers who supply those health care services. Projections of future Medicare expenditures and funding indicate that the program will place increasing financial demands on the federal budget and on beneficiaries over time. In response to these concerns, Congress may consider a range of

Medicare reform options, from making changes within the current structure, including modifying provider payments and revising existing oversight and regulatory mechanisms, to redesigning the entire program.

The Committees of jurisdiction for the entitlement (or benefits) portion of Medicare are the Senate Committee on Finance, the House Committee on Ways and Means, and the House Committee on Energy and Commerce. The House and Senate Committees on Appropriations have jurisdiction over the discretionary spending used to administer and oversee the program.

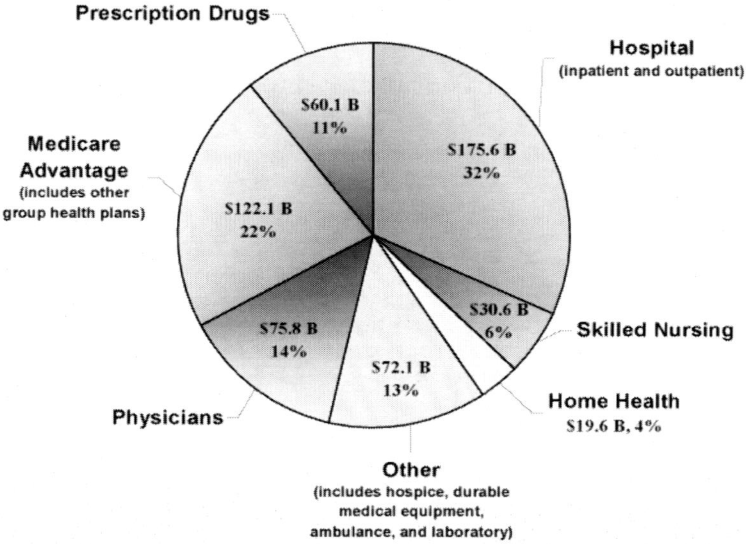

Source: Figure by CRS based on data from the Congressional Budget Office, March 2012 Medicare Baseline.

Note: The $555.9 billion for benefit payments does not include administration costs or recoveries.

Figure 1. Projected Medicare Benefit Spending, by Category, FY2012; ($555.9 billion).

Medicare History

Medicare was enacted in 1965 (P.L. 89-97) in response to the concern that only about half of the nation's seniors had health insurance, and most of those had coverage only for inpatient hospital costs. The new program, which became effective July 1, 1966, included Part A coverage for hospital and post-hospital services and Part B coverage for doctors and other medical services. As is the case for the Social Security program, Part A is financed by payroll taxes levied on current workers and their employers; persons must pay into the system for 40 calendar quarters to become entitled to premium-free benefits. Medicare Part B is voluntary, with a monthly premium required of beneficiaries who choose to enroll. Payments to health care providers under both Part A and Part B were originally based on the most common form of payment at the time, namely "reasonable costs" for hospital and other institutional services or "usual, customary and reasonable charges" (UCR)[1] for physicians and other medical services.

Medicare is considered a social insurance program and is the second largest such federal program, after Social Security. The 1965 law also established Medicaid, the federal/state health insurance program for the poor; this was an expansion of previous welfare-based assistance programs. Some low-income individuals qualify for both Medicare and Medicaid.

In the ensuing years, Medicare has undergone considerable change. P.L. 92-603, enacted in 1972, expanded program coverage to certain individuals under 65 (the disabled and persons with end-stage renal disease (ESRD)),[2] and introduced managed care into Medicare by allowing private insurance entities to provide Medicare benefits in exchange for a monthly capitated payment. This law also began to place limitations on the definitions of reasonable costs and charges in order to gain some control over program spending which, even initially, exceeded original projections.

During the 1980s and 1990s, a number of laws were enacted that included provisions designed to further stem the rapid increase in program spending through modifications to the way payments to providers were determined, and to postpone the insolvency of the Medicare Part A trust fund. This was typically achieved through tightening rules governing payments to providers of services and limiting the annual updates in such payments. The program moved from payments based on reasonable costs and reasonable charges to payment systems under which a predetermined payment amount was established for a specified unit of service. At the same time, beneficiaries were given expanded options to obtain covered services through private managed care arrangements, typically health maintenance organizations (HMOs). Most Medicare payment provisions were incorporated into larger budget reconciliation bills designed to control overall federal spending.

This effort culminated in the enactment of the Balanced Budget Act of 1997 (BBA 97, P.L. 105- 33). This law slowed the rate of growth in payments to providers and established new payment systems for certain categories of providers. It also established the Medicare+Choice program, which expanded private plan options for beneficiaries and changed the way most of these plans were paid. BBA 97 further expanded preventive services covered by the program.

Subsequently, Congress became concerned that the BBA 97 cuts in payments to providers were somewhat larger than originally anticipated. Therefore, legislation was enacted in both 1999 (Balanced Budget Refinement Act of 1999, BBRA, P.L. 106-113) and 2000 (Medicare, Medicaid, and SCHIP Benefits Improvement and Protection Act of 2000, BIPA, P.L. 106-554) to mitigate the impact of BBA 97 on providers.

In 2003, Congress enacted the Medicare Prescription Drug, Improvement, and Modernization Act of 2003 (MMA, P.L. 108-173),[3] which included a major benefit expansion and placed increasing emphasis on the private sector to deliver and manage benefits. The MMA included provisions that (1) created a new voluntary outpatient prescription drug benefit to be administered by private entities; (2) replaced the Medicare+Choice program with the Medicare Advantage (MA) program and raised payments to plans in order to increase their availability for beneficiaries; (3) introduced the concept of income testing into Medicare, with higher-income persons paying larger Part B premiums beginning in 2007; (4) modified some provider payment rules; (5) expanded covered preventive services; and (6) created a specific process for overall program review if general revenue spending exceeded a specified threshold.

During the 109th Congress, two laws were enacted that incorporated minor modifications to Medicare's payment rules. These were the Deficit Reduction Act of 2005 (DRA, P.L. 109-171) and the Tax Relief and Health Care Act of 2006 (TRHCA, P.L. 109-432). In the 110th Congress, additional changes were incorporated in the Medicare, Medicaid, and SCHIP Extension Act of 2007 (MMSEA, P.L. 110-173)[4] and the Medicare Improvements for Patients and Providers Act of 2008 (MIPPA, P.L. 110-275).[5]

In the 111th Congress, comprehensive health reform legislation was enacted that, among other things, made statutory changes to the Medicare program. The Patient Protection and Affordable Care Act (ACA; P.L. 111-148), enacted on March 23, 2010, included numerous provisions affecting Medicare payments, payment rules, covered benefits, and the delivery of care. The Health Care and Education Affordability Reconciliation Act of 2010 (the Reconciliation Act, or HCERA; P.L. 111-152), enacted on March 30, 2010, made changes to a number of Medicare-related provisions in the ACA and added several new provisions.[6] Included in the ACA, as amended, are provisions that (1) constrain Medicare's annual payment increases for certain providers; (2) change payment rates in the Medicare Advantage program so that they more closely resemble those in fee-for-service; (3) reduce payments to hospitals that serve a large number of low-income patients; (4) create an Independent Payment Advisory Board that will make recommendations to adjust Medicare payment rates; (5) phase out the Part D prescription drug benefit "doughnut hole"; (6) increase resources and enhance activities to prevent fraud and abuse; and (7) provide incentives to increase the quality and efficiency of care, such as creating value-based purchasing programs for certain types of providers, allowing accountable care organizations (ACOs) that meet certain quality and efficiency standards to share in the savings,[7] creating a voluntary pilot program that bundles payments for physician, hospital, and post-acute care services, and adjusting payments to hospitals for readmissions related to certain potentially preventable conditions.

During the first session of the 112th Congress, on August 2, 2011, the Budget Control Act of 2011 (BCA; P.L. 112-25) was enacted. It provided for increases in the debt limit and established procedures designed to reduce the federal budget deficit, including the creation of a Joint Select Committee on Deficit Reduction.[8] The failure of the Joint Committee to propose budget reduction legislation by its mandated deadline triggered automatic spending reductions ("sequestration") in years 2013 through 2021. Unless Congress takes action to prevent these cuts, most Medicare program expenditures will be subject to reductions of up to 2% in each of those years.[9] Under sequestration, Medicare's benefit structure would generally remain unchanged; however, most Medicare plans and providers would see a reduction in their Medicare payments. Spending for certain Medicare payments are exempt from sequestration and would therefore not be reduced. These exemptions include (1) Part D low-income subsidies, (2) the Part D catastrophic subsidy, and (3) Qualified Individual (QI) premiums. Some Medicare administrative and operational expenditures could be subject to reductions higher than 2%.[10] CBO estimates that Medicare spending reductions will total approximately $123 billion over nine years.[11]

Eligibility and Enrollment

Most persons aged 65 or older are automatically entitled to premium-free Part A because they or their spouse paid Medicare payroll taxes for at least 40 quarters (10 years) on earnings covered by either the Social Security or the

Railroad Retirement systems. Persons under age 65 who receive cash disability benefits from Social Security or the Railroad Retirement systems for at least 24 months are also entitled to Part A. (Since there is a five-month waiting period for cash payments, the Medicare waiting period is effectively 29 months.)[12] The 24-month waiting period is waived for persons with amyotrophic lateral sclerosis (ALS, "Lou Gehrig's disease"). Individuals of any age with ESRD who receive dialysis on a regular basis or a kidney transplant are eligible for Medicare. Medicare coverage for individuals with ESRD usually starts the first day of the fourth month of dialysis treatments. In addition, individuals with one or more specified lung diseases or types of cancer who lived for six months during a specified period prior to diagnosis in an area subject to a public health emergency declaration by the Environmental Protection Agency (EPA) as of June 17, 2009, are also deemed entitled to benefits under Part A and eligible to enroll in Part B.

Persons over age 65 who are not automatically entitled to Part A may obtain coverage by paying a monthly premium ($451 in 2012) or, for persons with at least 30 quarters of covered employment, a reduced monthly premium ($248 in 2012). In addition, disabled persons who lose their cash benefits solely because of higher earnings, and subsequently lose their extended Medicare coverage, may continue their Medicare enrollment by paying a premium, subject to limitations.

Generally, enrollment in Medicare Part B is voluntary. All persons entitled to Part A (and persons over 65 not entitled to premium-free Part A) may enroll in Part B by paying a monthly premium. For most Part B enrollees, the 2012 monthly premium is $99.90.[13] (See the "Part B" section, below.) While enrollment in Part B is voluntary for most individuals, in most cases, those who voluntarily enroll in Part A must also enroll in Part B. Additionally, ESRD beneficiaries and Medicare Advantage enrollees (discussed below) must also enroll in Part B.

Together, Parts A and B of Medicare comprise "original Medicare," which covers benefits on a fee-for-service (FFS) basis. Beneficiaries have another option for coverage through private plans, called the Medicare Advantage (MA or Part C) program. When beneficiaries first become eligible for Medicare, they may chose either original Medicare or they may enroll in a private MA plan. Each fall, there is an annual open enrollment period during which time Medicare beneficiaries may choose a different MA plan, or leave or join the MA program.[14] Beneficiaries are to receive information about their options to help them make informed decisions.[15] In 2012, the annual open enrollment period will be from October 15 to December 7 for plan choices starting the following January. Starting in 2012, MA plans with a 5-star quality rating will be allowed to enroll Medicare beneficiaries who are either in traditional Medicare or in an MA plan with a lower quality rating at any time.

Finally, each individual enrolled in either Part A or Part B is also entitled to obtain qualified prescription drug coverage through enrollment in a Part D prescription drug plan. Similar to Part B, enrollment in Part D is voluntary and the beneficiary pays a monthly premium. Beginning in 2011, some higher-income enrollees pay higher premiums, similar to enrollees in Part B. Generally, beneficiaries enrolled in an MA plan providing qualified prescription drug coverage (MA-PD plan) must obtain their prescription drug coverage through that plan.[16]

In general, individuals who do not enroll in Part B or Part D during an initial enrollment period (when they first become eligible for Medicare) must pay a permanent penalty of increased monthly premiums if they choose to enroll at a later date. Individuals who do not enroll in Part B during their initial enrollment period may enroll only during the annual open enrollment period, which occurs from January 1–March 31 each year. Coverage begins the following July 1. However, the law waives the Part B late enrollment penalty for current workers who have primary coverage through their own or a spouse's employer-sponsored plan. These individuals have a special enrollment period once their employment ends; as long as they enroll in Part B during this time, they will not be subject to penalty.

Individuals who do not enroll in Part D during their initial enrollment period may enroll during the annual open enrollment period, which corresponds with the Part C annual enrollment period—from October 15 to December 7, with coverage effective the following January. Individuals are not subject to the Part D penalty if they have maintained "creditable" drug coverage through another source, such as retiree health coverage offered by a former employer or union. However, once employees retire or have no access to "creditable" Part D coverage, a penalty will apply unless they sign up for coverage during a special enrollment period. Finally, for persons who qualify for the low-income subsidy for Part D, the delayed-enrollment penalty does not apply.

Benefits and Payments

Medicare Parts A, B, and D each cover different services, with Part C providing a private plan alternative for Medicare services, except hospice. The

Parts A-D covered services are described below, along with a description of Medicare's payments.

Part A

Part A provides coverage for inpatient hospital services, post-hospital skilled nursing facility (SNF) services, home health services, and hospice care, subject to certain conditions and limitations. Approximately 17% of Part A enrollees use Part A services during a year.

Inpatient Hospital Services

Medicare inpatient hospital services include (1) bed and board; (2) nursing services; (3) use of hospital facilities; (4) drugs, biologics, supplies, appliances, and equipment; and (5) diagnostic and therapeutic items and services. (Physicians' services provided during an inpatient stay are paid under the physician fee schedule and discussed below in the "Physicians and Non-physician Practitioner Services" section.) Coverage for inpatient services is linked to an individual's benefit period or "spell of illness" (defined as beginning on the day a patient enters a hospital and ending when he or she has not been in a hospital or SNF for 60 days). An individual admitted to a hospital more than 60 days after the last discharge from a hospital or SNF begins a new benefit period. Coverage in each benefit period is subject to the following conditions:

- Days 1-60. Beneficiary pays a deductible ($1,156 in 2012).
- Days 61-90. Beneficiary pays a *daily* coinsurance charge ($289 in 2012).
- Days 91-150. After 90 days, the beneficiary may draw on one or more of 60 lifetime reserve days, provided they have not been previously used. (Each of the 60 lifetime reserve days can be used only once during an individual's lifetime.) For lifetime reserve days, the beneficiary pays a daily coinsurance charge ($578 in 2012); otherwise the beneficiary pays all costs.
- Days 151 and over. Beneficiary pays for all costs for these days.

Inpatient mental health care in a psychiatric facility is limited to 190 days during a patient's lifetime. Cost sharing is structured similarly to that for stays in a general hospital (above).

Medicare makes payments to most acute care hospitals under the inpatient prospective payment (IPPS) system, using a prospectively determined amount for each discharge. Medicare's payments to hospitals is the product of two components: (1) a discharge payment amount adjusted by a wage index for the area where the hospital is located or where it has been reclassified, and (2) the weight associated with the Medicare severity-diagnosis related group (MS-DRG) to which the patient is assigned. This weight reflects the relative costliness of the average patient in that MS-DRG, which is revised annually, generally effective October 1 of each year.

Additional payments are made to hospitals for cases with extraordinary costs (outliers), indirect costs incurred by teaching hospitals for graduate medical education, and disproportionate share hospital (DSH) payments to those hospitals serving a certain volume of low-income patients. Additional payments may also be made for qualified new technologies that have been approved for special add-on payments. In FY2012, certain low volume hospitals will receive an add-on payment for each Medicare discharge, an amount that ranges from 25% for hospitals with less than 200 Medicare discharges to no adjustment for hospitals with more than 1,600 Medicare discharges. Prospective payments are also made for inpatient capital costs.

Medicare also makes payments outside the IPPS system for direct costs associated with graduate medical education (GME) for hospital residents, subject to certain limits. In addition, Medicare reimburses hospitals for 70% of the allowable costs associated with beneficiaries' unpaid deductible and copayment amounts as well as for the costs for certain other services.

Additional payments or special treatment may apply for hospitals meeting one of the following designations: (1) sole community hospitals (SCHs), (2) Medicare dependent hospitals, and (3) rural referral centers. Certain hospitals or distinct hospital units are exempt from IPPS and paid on an alternative basis,[17] including (1) inpatient rehabilitation facilities, (2) long-term care hospitals, (3) psychiatric facilities including hospitals and distinct part units, (4) children's hospitals and cancer hospitals, and (5) critical access hospitals.

Skilled Nursing Facility (SNF) Services

Medicare covers up to 100 days of post-hospital care for persons needing skilled nursing or rehabilitation services on a daily basis.[18] The SNF stay must be preceded by an inpatient hospital stay of at least three days, and the transfer to the SNF typically must occur within 30 days of the hospital discharge. There is no beneficiary cost-sharing for the first 20 days of a Medicare-covered SNF stay. For days 21 to 100 beneficiaries are subject to daily coinsurance charges ($144.50 in 2012). The 100-day limit begins again with a new spell of illness.

SNF services are paid under a prospective payment system (PPS), which is based on a per diem urban or rural base payment rate, adjusted for case mix (average severity of illness) and area wages. The per diem rate generally covers all services, including room and board, provided to the patient that day. The case-mix adjustment is made using the resource utilization groups (RUGs) classification system, which uses patient assessments to assign a beneficiary to one of 66 groups that reflect the beneficiary's expected use of services. Patient assessments are done at various times during a patient's stay and the RUG category a beneficiary is placed in can change with changes in the beneficiary's condition. Extra payments are not made for extraordinarily costly cases ("outliers").

Home Health Services

Medicare covers visits by participating home health agencies for beneficiaries who (1) are confined to home, (2) need skilled nursing care on an intermittent basis, or (3) need physical or occupational therapy or speech language therapy. After establishing such eligibility, the continuing need for occupational therapy services may extend the eligibility period. Covered services include part-time or intermittent nursing care, physical or occupational therapy or speech language pathology services, medical social services, home health aide services, and medical supplies and durable medical equipment. The services must be provided under a plan of care established by a physician, and the plan must be reviewed by the physician at least every 60 days.

Home health services are covered under both Medicare Parts A and B. Part A covers up to 100 visits following a stay in a hospital or SNF. Part A also covers all home health services for persons not enrolled in Part B. All other home health services are covered under Part B. There is no beneficiary cost-sharing for home health services (though some other Part B services provided in connection with the visit, such as durable medical equipment, are subject to cost-sharing charges).

Home health services are paid under a home health PPS, based on 60-day episodes of care; a patient may have an unlimited number of episodes. Under the PPS, a nationwide base payment amount is adjusted by differences in wages (using the hospital wage index). This amount is then adjusted for case mix using the applicable Home Health Resource Group (HHRG) to which the beneficiary has been assigned. The HHRG applicable to a beneficiary is determined following an assessment of the patient's condition and care needs using the Outcome and Assessment Information Set (OASIS); there are 153 HHRGs. Further payment adjustments may be made for outlier visits (for extremely costly patients), a significant change in a beneficiary's condition, a partial episode which occurs because a beneficiary transfers from one agency to another, a low utilization adjustment for beneficiaries receiving four or fewer visits, or an agency's failure to submit quality data to CMS.

Hospice Care

The Medicare hospice benefit covers services designed to provide palliative care and management of a terminal illness; the benefit includes drugs and medical and support services. These services are provided to Medicare beneficiaries with a life expectancy of six months or less for two 90-day periods, followed by an unlimited number of 60-day periods. The individual's attending physician and the hospice physician must certify the need for the first benefit period, but only the hospice physician needs to recertify for subsequent periods. Starting January 1, 2011, a hospice physician or nurse practitioner must have a face-to-face encounter with the individual to determine continued eligibility prior to the 180th day recertification, and for each subsequent recertification. Hospice care is provided in lieu of most other Medicare services related to the curative treatment of the terminal illness. Beneficiaries electing hospice care from a hospice program may receive curative services for illnesses or injuries unrelated to their terminal illness and they may disenroll from the hospice at any time. Nominal cost-sharing is required for drugs and respite care.

Payment for hospice care is based on one of four prospectively determined rates (which correspond to four different levels of care) for each day a beneficiary is under the care of the hospice. The four rate categories are routine home care, continuous home care, inpatient respite care, and general inpatient care. Payment rates are adjusted to reflect differences in area wage levels, using the hospital wage index.[19] Payments to a hospice are subject to an aggregate cap that limits the average per beneficiary cost to a cap that is adjusted annually by changes to the medical care expenditure category of the Consumer Price Index for all urban consumers (CPI-U).

Part A Services for End-Stage Renal Disease (ESRD)

Individuals with ESRD are eligible for all services covered under Parts A and B. Kidney transplantation services, to the extent they are inpatient hospital services, are subject to the inpatient hospital PPS. However, kidney acquisition costs are paid on a reasonable cost basis. (See "Part B Services for End-Stage Renal Disease" for an explanation of dialysis benefits and payments, as well as other Part B ESRD services.)

Part B

Medicare Part B covers physicians' services, outpatient hospital services, durable medical equipment, and other medical services. Initially, over 98% of the eligible population voluntarily enrolled in Part B, but in recent years, the percentage has fallen to about 93%.[20] Over 70% of Part B enrollees use Part B services during a year. The program generally pays 80% of the approved amount (most commonly, a fee schedule or other predetermined amount) for covered services in excess of the annual deductible ($140 in 2012). The beneficiary is liable for the remaining 20%.

Most providers and practitioners are subject to limits on amounts they can bill beneficiaries for covered services. For example, physicians and some other practitioners may choose whether or not to accept "assignment" on a claim. When a physician accepts assignment, the physician can only bill the beneficiary the 20% coinsurance plus any unmet deductible. When a physician agrees to accept assignment on all Medicare claims in a given year, the physician is referred to as a "participating physician." There are several advantages to being a participating provider, including higher reimbursement under the Medicare fee schedule, a lower beneficiary copayment, and automatic forwarding of Medigap claims.

Physicians who do not agree to accept assignment on all Medicare claims in a given year are referred to as nonparticipating physicians. Nonparticipating physicians may or may not accept assignment for a given service. If they do not, they may charge beneficiaries more than the fee schedule amount on nonassigned claims; however, these "balance billing" charges are subject to certain limits. Alternatively, physicians may choose not to accept any Medicare payment and enter into private contracts with their patients.

For some providers, such as nurse practitioners and physician assistants, assignment is mandatory; these providers can only bill the beneficiary the 20% coinsurance and any unmet deductible. For other Part B services, such as durable medical equipment, assignment is optional; for these services, applicable providers may bill beneficiaries for amounts above Medicare's recognized payment level and may do so without limit.[21]

Physicians and Non-physician Practitioner Services

Medicare Part B covers medically necessary doctors' services, outpatient care, home health services, some preventive care, and some other medical services. Certain limitations apply for services provided by chiropractors and podiatrists. Beneficiary cost-sharing is typically 20% of the approved amount, although preventive care services require no coinsurance from the beneficiary and outpatient mental health services are currently in the third of a five-year phase-in that will reduce beneficiary responsibility from 50% to 20% by 2014.[22] Covered non-physician practitioner services include, but are not limited to, those provided by physician assistants, nurse practitioners, certified registered nurse anesthetists, and clinical social workers.

A number of Part B services are paid under the physician fee schedule. These include services of physicians, non-physician practitioners, and therapists. Most services described below are paid under the physician fee schedule. There are over 7,000 service codes under the fee schedule.

The fee schedule assigns relative values to each service code. These relative values reflect physician work (based on time, skill, and intensity involved), practice expenses, and malpractice expenses. The relative values are adjusted for geographic variations in the costs of practicing medicine. These geographically adjusted relative values are converted into a dollar payment amount by a national conversion factor. The conversion factor is updated each year by a formula specified in law. The update percentage is based on the Medicare Economic Index (MEI, which measures changes in the prices of the inputs required to provide physician services) subject to an adjustment to match spending under the sustainable growth rate (SGR) system, which establishes a target for total cumulative expenditures since 1996. If total expenditures exceed the target, the update for a future year is reduced. Application of the SGR formula would have led to negative updates each year since 2002. However, Congress has acted several times to avert reductions, thereby overriding the statutory formula for the 2003-2012 period. The update to the conversion factor was 0% (compared to 2009 payment levels) for January through May 2010 and 2.2% for June 2010 through December 2011.[23] The fee schedule payments will be maintained at this level through 2012.[24]

In addition to the fee schedule reimbursements, physicians who report on selected quality measures for services for which quality measures are established will receive bonus payments for those services provided beginning in July 2007. The bonus payments were 1.5% during the second half of 2007 and for 2008, 2.0% for 2009 and 2010, 1.0% for 2011, and 0.5% in 2012. The bonus remains at 0.5% in 2013 and 2014 for those who successfully report the measures. Subsequently, those providers who fail to successfully report the measures will be subject to a 1.5% penalty in 2015 and a 2% penalty in 2016 and future years. Additional bonus payments will be made for 2009-2013 for Medicare professionals providing covered services who are successful electronic prescribers and in 2011-2014 for those who meet the requirements of a Maintenance of Certification Program (MOCP).[25]

Therapy Services

Medicare therapy services include physical therapy, occupational therapy, and speech language pathology services. The program establishes annual limits (therapy caps) on covered services. The first is a $1,880 per beneficiary annual cap in 2012 for all outpatient physical therapy services and speech language pathology services. The second is a $1,880 per beneficiary annual cap in 2012 for all outpatient occupational therapy services. The limits, which are updated annually, apply to services provided by independent therapists as well as to those provided by comprehensive outpatient rehabilitation facilities (CORFs) and other rehabilitation agencies. The Secretary is required to implement an exceptions process, effective from 2006 through 2011, for services meeting specified criteria for medically necessary services. The limits do not apply to outpatient services provided by hospitals.

Preventive Services

The original Medicare statutes prohibited payment for covered items and services that are "not reasonable and necessary for the diagnosis or treatment of illness or injury or to improve the functioning of a malformed body member," which effectively excluded preventive and screening services.[26] In recent years, Congress has added and expanded Medicare coverage for a number of such services through legislation, including MMA, MIPPA, and ACA. Under current law, if a preventive service is recommended for use by the U.S. Preventive Services Task Force (USPSTF, an independent evidence-review panel)[27] and Medicare covers the service, all cost-sharing must be waived. Also, the HHS Secretary may add coverage of a USPSTF-recommended service that is not already covered. Coverage for preventive and screening services currently includes, among other services: (1) a "welcome to Medicare" physical exam during the first year of enrollment in Part B and an annual visit and prevention plan thereafter; (2) flu vaccine (annual), pneumococcal vaccine, and hepatitis B vaccine (for persons at high risk); (3) screening tests for breast, cervical, prostate, and colorectal cancers; (4) screening for other conditions such as depression, heart disease, glaucoma, and osteoporosis; and (5) intensive behavioral therapy for heart disease and for obesity.[28] These services are covered under the Medicare Part B fee schedule.

Clinical Lab and other Diagnostic Tests

Part B covers clinical laboratory tests. Neither copayment nor deductible applies to services paid under the Medicare clinical laboratory fee schedule. There is no coinsurance for clinical laboratory services. Clinical lab services are paid on the basis of area-wide fee schedules. There is a ceiling on payment amounts equal to 74% of the median of all fee schedules for the test. In general, annual increases in clinical lab fees are based on the percentage change in the CPI-U. However, Congress has modified the update in recent years, by (1) freezing the fee schedule amounts through 2008 and (2) reducing the update that would otherwise apply by 0.5 percentage points each year, for 2009-2013.

Part B also covers diagnostic x-ray tests and other diagnostic tests, as well as x-ray, radium, and radioisotope therapy. Generally, these services are paid for under the physician fee schedule.

Durable Medical Equipment, Prosthetics, Orthotics and Supplies (DMEPOS)

Medicare covers a wide variety of equipment and devices under the heading of durable medical equipment (DME), and prosthetics, orthotics (PO) if they are medically necessary and are prescribed by a physician. DME is defined as equipment that (1) can withstand repeated use, (2) is used primarily to serve a medical purpose, (3) is not generally useful in the absence of an illness or injury, and (4) is appropriate for use in the home. DME includes such items as hospital beds, wheelchairs, blood glucose monitors, and oxygen and oxygen equipment. It also includes related supplies, such as drugs and biologics that are necessary for the effective use of the product. PO is defined as items that replace all or part of a body organ, such as colostomy bags and pacemakers, as well as leg, arm, back, and neck braces and artificial legs, arms, and eyes. Medicare also covers some items or supplies (S), such as disposable surgical dressings that do not meet the definitions of DME or PO.

Except in competitive bidding areas (described below), Medicare pays for most DMEPOS based on fee schedules. Medicare pays 80% of the lower of the supplier's charge for the item or the fee schedule amount. The beneficiary is responsible for the remaining 20%. In general, fee schedule amounts are updated each year by a (1) measure of price inflation, and (2) a measure of economy-wide productivity, which may result in lower fee schedule amounts from one year to the nest. In addition, Congress has specified a reduction or elimination in the price inflation updates in recent years.

Numerous studies and investigations have shown that Medicare pays more for certain items of DME and PO than some other health insurers and some retail outlets.[29] Such overpayments may be due partly to the fee schedule mechanism of payment. MMA required the Secretary to establish a Competitive Acquisition Program for certain DMEPOS in specified areas. Instead of paying for medical equipment based on a fee schedule established by law, payment for items in competitive bidding areas is based on the supplier bids. MIPPA delayed the program and required the first round of the program to be re-bid, in addition to other changes. The re-bid took place in 2009 and the program started in nine metropolitan areas in January 2011.[30] The second round will expand the program to 91 additional areas. Bidding for round 2 began in January 2012, with payments based on those bids starting in July 2013.

Part B Drugs and Biologics[31]

Certain specified outpatient prescription drugs and biologics are covered under Medicare Part B. (However, most outpatient prescription drugs are covered under Part D, discussed below.) Covered Part B drugs and biologics include drugs furnished incident to physicians' services, immunosuppressive drugs following a Medicare-covered organ transplant, erythropoietin for treatment of anemia for persons with ESRD, oral anti-cancer drugs (provided they have the same active ingredients and are used for the same indications as chemotherapy drugs which would be covered if furnished incident to physicians services), and drugs needed for the effective use of DME. Generally, Medicare's reimbursement for Part B covered drugs equals 106% of the drug manufacturer's reported average sales price. Health care providers also receive a separate payment for administering Medicare Part B drugs. Medicare pays 80% of the amount paid to providers, while the beneficiaries are responsible for the remaining 20%.

Hospital Outpatient Department Services

Hospitals provide two distinct types of services to outpatients: services that are diagnostic in nature, and other services that aid the physician in the treatment of the patient. A hospital outpatient is a person who has not been admitted by the hospital as an inpatient but is registered on the hospital records as an outpatient. Generally, payments under the hospital outpatient prospective payment system (OPPS) cover the operating and capital-related costs that are directly related and integral to performing a procedure or furnishing a service on an outpatient basis. These payments cover services such as the use of an operating suite, treatment, procedure or recovery room; use of an observation bed as well as anesthesia; certain drugs or pharmaceuticals; incidental services; and other necessary or implantable supplies or services. Payments for services such as those provided by physicians and other professionals as well as therapy and clinical diagnostic laboratory services, among others, are separate.

Under the OPPS, the unit of payment for acute care hospitals is the individual service or procedure as assigned to an ambulatory payment classification (APC). To the extent possible, integral services and items (excluding physician services paid under the physician fee schedule) are bundled within each APC. Specified new technologies are assigned to "new technology APCs" until clinical and cost data are available to permit assignment into a "clinical APC."

Medicare's hospital outpatient payment is calculated by multiplying the relative weight associated with an APC by a conversion factor. For most APCs, 60% of the conversion factor is geographically adjusted by the wage index used for the inpatient prospective payment system. Except for new technology APCs, each APC has a relative weight that is based on the median cost of services in that APC. The OPPS also includes pass-through payments for new technologies (specific drugs, biologicals, and devices) and payments for outliers.[32]

Ambulatory Surgical Center Services

Medicare covers surgical and medical services performed in an ambulatory surgical center (ASC) that are (1) commonly performed on an inpatient basis but may be safely performed in an ASC; (2) not of a type that are commonly performed or that may be safely performed in physicians' offices; (3) limited to procedures requiring a dedicated operating room or suite and generally requiring a post-operative recovery room or short term (not overnight) convalescent room; and (4) not otherwise excluded from Medicare coverage.

Beginning in January 2008, Medicare pays for surgery-related facility services provided in ASCs using a payment system based on the OPPS. (Associated physician fees are paid for separately under the physician fee schedule.) Each of the 3,300 procedures approved for payment in an ASC is classified into an ambulatory payment classification (APC) group on the basis of clinical and cost similarity. The ASC system uses the same payment groups

(APCs) as the OPPS, and for most procedures, the same relative weights used in the OPPS also apply. The ASC system uses a conversion factor based on a percentage of the OPPS conversion factor. The percentage of this average dollar figure is set to ensure budget neutrality, so that total payments under the new ASC payment system should equal total payments under the old ASC payment system. A different payment method is used to set ASC payment for new, office-based procedures, separately payable drugs, and device-intensive procedures.[33] This policy also applies to separately payable radiology services. Separately payable drugs in an ASC are paid the same amount as if provided in a hospital outpatient department. Different rules apply for device intensive procedures (where a device that is packaged into an APC accounts for more than half of its total payments). Separate payments are made for corneal tissue acquisition, brachytherapy sources, certain radiology services, many drugs, and certain implantable devices.

Ambulance

Medicare Part B covers ambulance services to or from a hospital, critical access hospital, or a skilled nursing facility when other modes of transportation could endanger the Medicare beneficiary's health. Ambulance services must be provided by qualified suppliers, and are paid for on the basis of a fee schedule. The fee schedule establishes seven categories of ground ambulance services and two categories of air ambulance services. There is a national fee schedule for air ambulance services. For ground ambulance services, payments through 2009 were equal to the greater of the national fee schedule or a blend of 80% national and 20% regional fee schedule amounts. Beginning in 2010, the payments in all areas are based on the national fee schedule amount.

The payment for a service equals a base rate for the level of service plus payment for mileage, with geographic adjustments made to a portion of the base rate. Additionally, the base rate is increased for air ambulance trips originating in rural areas and mileage payments are increased for all trips originating in rural areas.

Rural Health Clinics and Federally Qualified Health Centers

Medicare covers Part B services in rural health clinics (RHCs) and federally qualified health centers (FQHCs) provided by (1) physicians and specified non-physician practitioners; (2) visiting nurses for homebound patients in home health shortage areas; (3) registered dieticians or nutritional professionals for diabetes training and medical nutrition therapy; and (4) others, as well as otherwise covered drugs.

RHCs and FQHCs are paid based on an "all-inclusive" rate per beneficiary visit subject to a per visit upper limit, adjusted annually for inflation.

Part B Services for End-Stage Renal Disease

Individuals with ESRD are eligible for all Part B Services. Part B also covers their dialysis services, drugs, biologicals (including erythropoiesis stimulating agents used in treating anemia as a result of ESRD), diagnostic laboratory tests, and other items and services furnished to individuals for the treatment of ESRD.

In effect since January 1, 2011, the new ESRD prospective payment system (PPS) makes no payment distinction as to the site where renal dialysis services are provided. With the implementation of the ESRD PPS, Medicare dialysis payments are bundled (phased in over four years, 2011 through 2014) using a single payment for Medicare renal dialysis services that includes (1) items and services included in the former payment system's base rate as of December 31, 2010; (2) erythropoiesis stimulating agents (ESAs) for the treatment of ESRD; (3) other drugs and biologicals for which payment was made separately (before bundling); and (4) diagnostic laboratory tests and other items and services furnished to individuals for the treatment of ESRD. The new system is case-mix adjusted based on factors such as patient weight, body mass index, comorbidities, length of time on dialysis, age, race, ethnicity, and other appropriate factors as determined by the Secretary of Health and Human Services. Dialysis facilities that fail to meet the performance standards of three ESRD-related quality measures receive reduced payments.

Part C, Medicare Advantage

Medicare Advantage (MA) is an alternative way for Medicare beneficiaries to receive covered benefits. Under MA, private health plans are paid a per-person amount to provide all Medicare covered benefits (except hospice) to beneficiaries who enroll in their plan. Medicare beneficiaries who are eligible for Part A, enrolled in Part B, and do not have ESRD are eligible to enroll in an MA plan if one is available in their area. Some MA plans may choose their service area (local MA plans), while others agree to serve one or more regions defined by the Secretary (regional MA plans). As of December

2011, nearly all Medicare beneficiaries had access to an MA plan and approximately 25% of beneficiaries were enrolled in one. Private plans may use different techniques to influence the medical care used by enrollees. Some plans, such as health maintenance organizations (HMOs), may require enrollees to receive care from a restricted network of medical providers; enrollees may be required to see a primary care physician who will coordinate their care and refer them to specialists as necessary. Other types of private plans, such as private fee-for-service (PFFS) plans, may look more like original Medicare, with fewer restrictions on the providers an enrollee can see and minimal coordination of care.

In general, MA plans offer additional benefits or require smaller co-payments or deductibles than original Medicare. Sometimes beneficiaries pay for these additional benefits through a higher monthly premium, but sometimes they are financed through plan savings. The extent of extra benefits and reduced cost-sharing varies by plan type and geography. However, Medicare Advantage plans are seen by some beneficiaries as an attractive alternative to more expensive supplemental insurance policies found in the private market.

By contract with CMS, a plan agrees to provide all required services covered in return for a capitated monthly payment adjusted for the demographics and health history of actually enrolled beneficiaries. The same monthly payment is made regardless of how many or few services a beneficiary actually uses. The plan is at-risk if costs, in the aggregate, exceed program payments; conversely, the plan can retain savings if aggregate costs are less than payments. Payments to MA plans are based on a comparison of each plan's estimated cost of providing Medicare covered services (a bid) relative to the maximum amount the federal government will pay for providing those services in the plan's service area (a benchmark). If a plan's bid is less than the benchmark, its payment equals its bid plus a rebate. Starting in 2012, the size of the rebate will be dependent on plan quality and will range from 50% to 70% of the difference between the bid and the benchmark. The rebate must be returned to enrollees in the form of either additional benefits, reduced cost-sharing, reduced Part B or Part D premiums, or some combination of these options. If a plan's bid is equal to or above the benchmark, its payment will be the benchmark amount and each enrollee in that plan will pay an additional premium, equal to the amount by which the bid exceeds the benchmark.

The MA benchmarks are determined through statutorily specified formulas that have changed over time. Since BBA 97, formulas have increased the benchmark amounts, in part, to encourage plan participation in all areas of the country. As a result, however, the benchmark amounts (and plan payments) in some areas are higher than the average cost of original FFS Medicare. Most recently, ACA changed the way benchmarks are to be calculated by tying them closer to (or below) spending in FFS Medicare, and adjusting them based on plan quality. At the time of passage, the Congressional Budget Office expected the ACA changes to result in reduced MA enrollment and plan subsidies for extra benefits, though the impact was expected to vary by market. Subsequently, the Secretary announced an MA plan quality demonstration to test whether different structures of bonus payments lead to greater quality improvements. The demonstration increases the size of the quality-adjusted benchmarks above levels authorized in the ACA, and expands the number of plans eligible to receive a quality-adjusted benchmarks. The demonstration may mitigate some of the reductions in enrollment and extra plan benefits that had been expected with the passage of the ACA.

In 2006, the MA program began to offer MA regional plans. Regional MA plans must agree to serve one or more regions designated by the Secretary. There are 26 MA regions consisting of states or groups of states. Regional plan benchmarks include two components: (1) a statutorily determined amount (comparable to benchmarks described above) and (2) a weighted average of plan bids. Thus, a portion of the benchmark is competitively determined. Similar to local plans, plans with bids below the benchmark are given a rebate, while plans with bids above the benchmark require an additional enrollee premium.

In general, MA eligible individuals may enroll in any MA plan that serves their area. However, some MA plans may restrict their enrollment to beneficiaries who meet additional criteria. For example, employer-sponsored MA plans are generally only available to the retirees of the company sponsoring the plan.

In addition, Medicare Special Needs Plans (SNPs) are a type of coordinated care MA plan that exclusively enrolls, or enrolls a disproportionate percentage of, special needs individuals. Special needs individuals are any MA eligible individuals who are either institutionalized as defined by the Secretary, eligible for both Medicare and Medicaid, or have a severe or disabling chronic condition and would benefit from enrollment in a specialized MA plan.

Part D

Medicare Part D provides coverage of outpatient prescription drugs to Medicare beneficiaries who choose to enroll in this optional benefit.[34] (As previously discussed, Part B provides limited coverage of some outpatient prescription drugs.) In 2011, about 60% of eligible Medicare beneficiaries enrolled in Part D. Prescription drug coverage is provided through private prescription drug plans (PDPs), which offer only prescription drug coverage, or through Medicare Advantage prescription drug plans (MA-PDs), which offer prescription drug coverage that is integrated with the health care coverage they provide to Medicare beneficiaries under Part C. Plans must meet certain minimum requirements; however, there are significant variations among them in benefit design, including differences in premiums, drugs included on plan formularies, and cost-sharing for particular drugs.

Qualified Part D prescription drug plans are required to offer either "standard coverage" or alternative coverage that has actuarially equivalent benefits. In 2012, "standard coverage" has a $320 deductible and a 25% coinsurance for costs between $320 and $2,930. From this point, there is minimal coverage until the beneficiary has out-of-pocket costs of $4,700 (about $6,657.50 in total spending); this coverage gap has been labeled the "doughnut hole." [35] Once the beneficiary reaches the catastrophic limit, the program pays all costs except for nominal cost-sharing. In 2010, Medicare sent a tax free, one-time $250 rebate check to each Part D enrollee who reached the doughnut hole. Starting in 2011, the coverage gap will be gradually reduced each year until it is eliminated in 2020.[36] In 2012, a 50% discount is provided by drug manufacturers for brand-name drugs and Medicare pays for 14% of the cost of generic drugs dispensed during the coverage gap. By 2020, through a combination of manufacturer discounts and increased Medicare coverage, Part D enrollees will be responsible for 25% of the costs in the coverage gap (the same as during the initial coverage period). Most plans offer actuarially equivalent benefits rather than the standard package, including alternatives such as reducing or eliminating the deductible, or using tiered cost-sharing with lower cost-sharing for generic drugs.

Medicare's payments to plans are determined through a competitive bidding process, and enrollee premiums are tied to plan bids. Plans are paid a risk-adjusted monthly per capita amount based on their bids during a given plan year. Part D plan sponsors determine payments for drugs and are expected to negotiate prices. The federal government is prohibited from interfering in the price negotiations between drug manufacturers, pharmacies, and plans (the so-called "non-interference clause").

Part D also provides enhanced coverage for low-income enrolled individuals, such as persons who previously received drug benefits under Medicaid (known as "dual eligibles"—enrollees in both Medicare and Medicaid). Additionally, certain persons who do not qualify for Medicaid, but whose incomes are below 150% of poverty, may also receive assistance for some portion of their premium and cost-sharing charges.

MMA included significant incentives for employers to continue to offer coverage to their retirees by providing a 28% federal subsidy. In 2012, the maximum potential subsidy per covered retiree is $1,730.40 for employers or unions offering drug coverage that is at least actuarially equivalent (called "creditable" coverage), to standard coverage.[37] Employers or unions may select an alternative option (instead of taking the subsidy) with respect to Part D, such as electing to pay a portion of the Part D premiums. They may also elect to provide enhanced coverage, though this has some financial consequences for the employer or union. Alternatively, employers or unions may contract with a PDP or MA-PD to offer the coverage or become a Part D plan sponsor themselves for their retirees.

Administration

At the federal level, Medicare is administered by CMS within the Department of Health and Human Services (HHS). CMS contracts with private entities to administer much of the program's day-to-day activities. Functions such as paying providers (processing reimbursement claims), enrolling providers and suppliers in Medicare, educating providers about billing requirements, and processing appeals are performed by Medicare Administrative Contractors (MACs). MMA required the Secretary to implement FFS contracting reform by 2011. CMS completed Round I of Parts A and B FFS contractor reform by awarding contracts to 15 A/B MACs to process Part A and B claims and four DME MACs to process DME supplier claims. CMS plans to further consolidate A/B MACs to 10 contracts during a second round of contract awards, which began in July 2010.[38]

Under authority provided in the Health Insurance Portability and Accountability Act of 1996 (HIPAA, P.L. 104-191), CMS contracts with private organizations to protect Medicare trust funds from making improper payments and from fraud and abuse.[39] In addition, to reducing improper

Medicare payments, CMS contracts with other private entities, called Recovery Audit Contractors (RACs). In MMA, Congress authorized a three-year demonstration to test RACs, but has since expanded RACs nationwide and applied them to all parts of Medicare. RACs are responsible for reducing Medicare's improper payment rates by identifying underpayments and overpayments made to providers, recovering overpayments, and working with providers to prevent future improper payments. RACs are paid a contingency fee based on a percentage of the overpayments they recover from Medicare providers and suppliers. In FY2010, the Medicare RAC program identified approximately $92 million in FFS claims corrections, of which $75 million was overpayments and $17 million was underpayments. In FY2011, the Medicare RAC program identified $939 million in FFS corrections, $797 million in overpayments and $142 million in underpayments.[40]

In addition to Medicare program integrity enhancements in ACA, Section 4241 of the Small Business and Jobs Act of 2010 (SBJA, P.L. 111-240) appropriated $100 million for CMS to initiate predictive modeling and other analytics technologies ("predictive analytics technologies").[41] Predictive analytics technologies have been compared to technologies used in private sector financial services industries, such as banking, insurance, and credit cards, to reduce fraudulent billing. By combining data and information from multiple sources, including Medicare FFS claims history (aberrant billing patterns), enrollment information, background checks, and other public and private information (links to questionable affiliations), complaints, predictive analytics technologies could help to determine if claims were legitimate before they were paid.

Medicare's quality assurance activities are handled by state Survey Agencies and Quality Improvement Organizations (QIOs), which operate in all states, the District of Columbia, Puerto Rico, and the U.S. Virgin Islands. State survey agencies are responsible for inspecting Medicare provider facilities (i.e., nursing homes, home health agencies, and hospitals) to ensure they are in compliance with federal safety and quality standards referred to as Conditions of Participation. QIOs monitor the quality of care delivered to Medicare beneficiaries and educate providers on the latest quality improvement techniques.

In January 2011, CMS established a Center for Medicare and Medicaid Innovation (CMI).[42] The purpose of CMI is to test and evaluate innovative payment and service delivery models to reduce program expenditures under Medicare, Medicaid, and the State Children's Health Insurance Program (CHIP) while preserving or enhancing the quality of care furnished under these programs. In selecting the models, the Secretary is required to give preference to those that improve the coordination, quality, and efficiency of health care services.

Financing

Medicare's financial operations are accounted for through two trust funds, the Hospital Insurance (HI) trust fund for Part A and the Supplementary Medical Insurance (SMI) trust fund for Part B, which are maintained by the Department of the Treasury. The HI and SMI trust funds are overseen by a board of trustees that makes annual reports to Congress. HI is primarily funded by payroll taxes, while SMI is funded through general revenue transfers and premiums.[43]

The trust funds are simply accounting mechanisms; there is no actual transfer of money into and out of a fund. Income to the trust funds is credited to the fund in the form of interest-bearing government securities. Expenditures for services and administrative costs are recorded against the fund. The securities represent obligations that the government has issued to itself. As long as the trust fund has a balance, the Treasury Department is authorized to make payments for it from the U.S. Treasury.

ACA established a new 15-member Independent Payment Advisory Board that will, beginning in 2014, make recommendations to reduce Medicare spending in years when Medicare costs are projected to exceed a target growth rate.[44] The board's proposals will take effect unless Congress passes an alternative measure that achieves the same level of savings. The board is prohibited from making proposals that ration care, raise taxes, increase Part B premiums, or change Medicare benefit, eligibility, or cost-sharing standards.

Part A Financing

The primary source of funding for Part A is payroll taxes paid by employees and employers. Each pays a tax of 1.45% on the employee's earnings; the self-employed pay 2.9%. Beginning in 2013, some higher-income employees will pay higher payroll taxes. Unlike Social Security, there is no upper limit on earnings subject to the tax. Other sources of income include (1) interest on federal securities held by the trust fund, (2) a portion of federal income taxes that individuals pay on their social security benefits, (3) premiums paid by voluntary enrollees who are not automatically entitled to Medicare Part A, (4) transfers from states, and (5) other revenues. Income for Part A is credited to the HI trust fund. Part A expenditures for CY2012 are estimated to reach approximately $270 billion.[45] About $208 billion of this amount is expected to be funded by payroll taxes and $34 billion by interest income and other sources; approximately $29 billion will need to be drawn out of accumulated assets in the HI trust fund to make up the difference between expected income and expenditures.

In 2008, Part A expenditures began to exceed payroll tax income; and, in 2009, the Medicare trustees estimated that the HI trust fund would become insolvent (i.e., have $0 in accumulated assets) by 2017. In 2010, subsequent to the enactment of health reform legislation, the Medicare Trustees estimated that changes made by ACA to reduce program spending and increase Part A revenues would extend the solvency of the HI trust fund for another 12 years, until 2029. Due mainly to a slower than expected economic recovery, the 2011 Medicare trustees report moved up the insolvency date by five years, to 2024. The 2012 report continues to project a 2024 insolvency date.[46]

Part B Financing

Medicare Part B is financed mostly from federal general revenues, with beneficiary premiums set at 25% of estimated program costs for the aged. (The disabled pay the same premium as the aged.) Income for Part B is credited to the SMI trust fund. Total spending for Part B is estimated to reach about $247 billion in CY2012, with general revenues financing approximately $166 billion of that amount.[47]

The 2012 monthly premium is $99.90 for most Medicare beneficiaries who voluntarily enroll in Part B.[48] Individuals receiving Social Security benefits have their Part B premium payments automatically deducted from their Social Security benefit checks. An individual's Social Security check cannot go down from one year to the next as a result of the annual Part B premium increase (except in the case of higher-income individuals subject to income-related premiums).

Since 2007, higher-income enrollees pay higher premiums. In 2012, individuals whose modified adjusted gross income (AGI) exceeds $85,000 and each member of a couple filing jointly whose modified AGI exceeds $170,000 are subject to higher premium amounts. These higher-income premiums range from 35% to 80% of the value of Part B, affecting about 4% of Medicare Part

B enrollees in 2012.[49] As a result of ACA, the income thresholds have been frozen at the 2010 level through 2019, which means that more people may be subject to the high-income premium over time.

Part C Financing

Payments for spending under the Medicare Advantage program are made in appropriate portions from the HI and SMI trust funds. There is no separate trust fund for Part C.

Part D Financing

Medicare Part D is financed through a combination of beneficiary premiums and federal general revenues. In addition, certain transfers are made from the states. These transfers, referred to as "clawback payments," represent a portion of the amounts states could otherwise have been expected to pay for drugs under Medicaid if drug coverage for the dual eligible population had not been transferred to Part D. Part D revenues are credited to a separate Part D account within the SMI trust fund. In CY2012, total spending for Part D is estimated to reach approximately $69 billion, with about $51 billion of that amount paid for by general revenues.[50]

In 2012, the base beneficiary premium is $31.08.[51] However, beneficiaries pay different premiums depending on the plan they have selected and whether they are entitled to low-income premium subsidies. Additionally, beginning in 2011, higher income Part D enrollees pay higher premiums. (The income thresholds are the same as for Part B, as described above.) On average, beneficiary premiums are set at 25.5% of expected total Part D costs for basic coverage.

Additional Insurance Coverage

While Medicare provides broad protection against the costs of many, primarily acute care, services, the program does not cover all services that may be used by its aged and disabled beneficiaries. For example, Medicare does not cover eyeglasses, hearing aids, dentures, or most long-term care services. Further, unlike most private insurance polices, it does not include an annual "catastrophic" cap on out-of-pocket spending on cost-sharing charges for services covered under Parts A and B (except for persons enrolled in Medicare Advantage plans).

Most Medicare beneficiaries have some coverage in addition to Medicare. The following are the main sources of additional coverage for Medicare enrollees.

- Medicare Advantage. Many MA plans offer services in addition to those covered under original Medicare, reduced cost sharing, or reduced Part B or D premiums. All MA plans have a catastrophic cap.[52]
- Employer Coverage. Coverage may be provided through a current or former employer. In recent years, a number of employers have cut back on the scope of retiree coverage. Some have dropped such coverage entirely, particularly for future retirees. As noted earlier, the MMA attempted to stem this trend, at least for prescription drug coverage, by offering subsidies to employers who offer drug coverage, at least as good as that available under Part D.
- Medigap. Individual insurance policies that supplement fee-for-service Medicare are referred to as Medigap policies. Beneficiaries with Medigap insurance typically have coverage for a portion of Medicare's deductibles and coinsurance; they may also have coverage for some items and services not covered by Medicare. Individuals select from a set of standardized plans, though not all plans are offered in all states.
- Medicaid. Certain low-income Medicare beneficiaries also may be eligible for full or partial benefits under their state's Medicaid program.[53] Individuals eligible for both Medicare and Medicaid are referred to as dual eligibles. The lowest-income dual eligibles qualify for full Medicaid benefits, so that the majority of their health care expenses are paid by either Medicare or Medicaid; Medicare pays first, with Medicaid picking up most of the remaining costs. In addition to full-benefit dual eligibles, state Medicaid programs pay Medicare premiums and some cost-sharing for other partial dual eligibles, who have higher income than full-benefit dual eligibles but are still considered to have low income.[54]
- Other Public Sources. Individuals may have additional coverage through the Department of Veterans Affairs, or TRICARE for military retirees eligible for Medicare (and enrolled in Part B).

In 2008, close to 90% of beneficiaries had some form of additional coverage. (Some persons may have had more than one type of additional coverage.)

Medicare Issues

Although recent health legislation helped to improve the financial outlook for Medicare, projected expenditures are still expected to outpace GDP growth and to consume an increasing portion of the federal budget. As such, the 112th Congress may continue to focus on Medicare spending as it considers ways to address the nation's growing deficit and debt. For example, the 112th Congress may consider the sustainability of reductions to providers' annual payment increases made by recent statutory changes, the potential impact of new delivery models to slow growth rates in medical expenditures and/or to improve quality, and the development of a viable long-term replacement for the current method of updating physician payments according to the sustainable growth rate (SGR) formula.

Some of the key policy issues and questions the second session of the 112th Congress may face include the following:

- A combination of factors have contributed to the rapid growth in Medicare spending. These include increases in overall medical costs driven by new and increasing use of technology and increases in the intensity and volume of services provided per beneficiary. While the percentage of the population over 65 and the life expectancy of the elderly has increased, these demographic effects have a secondary impact on spending compared to the increase in services per beneficiary. How will changes made in recent health care reform legislation affect the growth in Medicare expenditures and the long-term solvency of the Medicare Hospital Insurance (Part A) trust fund and the pressure on Part B premiums to rise? What will be the potential impact on the program if the BCA automatic spending reductions were to go into effect as required in 2013-2021? Will existing financing mechanisms be sufficient to support program spending over the long term? If not, what options are available to strengthen the program's financing and to ensure long-term sustainability?

- Under ACA, certain providers, such as hospitals, skilled nursing facilities (SNFs), and home health agencies (HHAs), face permanent reductions in the annual updates to their Medicare payment rates. Can, and if so, how will these providers modify service to become more efficient? Will Medicare payment reductions for these providers lead to higher prices to other payers or can increased efficiencies result in reduced costs to other payers as well? How will these reductions affect the availability of these services to Medicare beneficiaries? How may providers be affected by reduced payments under BCA sequestration requirements?
- Medicare payments to physicians and other providers continue to grow at rates that require ever-larger future reductions in the reimbursement rates under current law by the sustainable growth rate (SGR) system. Congress's continued reliance on short-term fixes to forestall reductions in the Medicare fee schedule prolongs the search for a long-term solution or replacement to the update formula. At the same time, each override becomes more costly. Additionally, uncertainty regarding the stability of Medicare's physician payments and the potential for future reductions has accelerated concern that Medicare beneficiaries will be increasingly unable to access providers should program participation fall as a result. Further, what will the impact be on Medicare beneficiary access to care due to increased demand for health care services as a result of ACA's Medicaid expansions and the expected growth in the number of insured in the private sector?
- A number of Medicare reimbursement policies affecting hospitals, skilled nursing facilities, ambulance services, and clinical laboratories are set to expire in 2012. These include such things as hospital inpatient Section 508 wage reclassifications, an extension of the exceptions process for outpatient therapy caps, hospital outpatient hold-harmless payments, and ambulance service add-on payments.[55] These policies have generally been extended each year over the past several years; the cost of extending these policies again through 2012 is expected to cost about $2.5 billion.[56] Congress will need to address whether these policies should be continued in both the short and long-term, and if so, it will need to determine how these extensions will be paid for.
- In 2012, almost all beneficiaries have the option to receive their Medicare covered benefits under the original Medicare program, or

through a private health plan under the Medicare Advantage (MA) program (also known as Medicare Part C). Prior to ACA, payments to MA plans exceeded the cost of original Medicare in many locations due to statutory payment rules designed to encourage plan availability. In recent years the number and type of plan choices have been high, however, the greater cost of these plans has been called into question. Starting in 2012, ACA changes how the maximum possible payments to MA plans are calculated, first by tying maximum payments closer to or below the level of spending in original Medicare and second, by adjusting payments based on plan quality. This may result in payment reductions for many MA plans. How will changes in MA payments affect plan availability and the types of supplemental benefits and reduced cost-sharing that some plans offer? Will the payment changes encourage higher plan quality or greater efficiency in the management and delivery of health care? Will a greater emphasis on plan quality encourage enrollees to switch to higher quality MA plans?

- Since 2011, pharmaceutical manufacturers have been required to provide a 50% discount on brand name drugs for enrollees in the coverage gap (often referred to as the "doughnut hole") in order to participate in the Medicare outpatient prescription drug (Part D) program. Additionally, the coverage gap is being gradually phased out and will be completely closed in 2020. How will the phaseout of the doughnut hole affect beneficiaries' out-of-pocket costs and their ability to access needed prescriptions? How many manufacturers will continue to provide 50% discounts for brand name drugs in the coverage gap? Will Medicare cover drugs that are medically necessary but whose manufacturers did not enter into an agreement to provide the discount? What will be the impact of the gap closure on total Medicare Part D expenditures and beneficiary premiums? What impact will the growing number of brand name drugs going off patent have on future Medicare Part D program and enrollee expenditures?
- Medicare cost-sharing is generally higher than it is under private employer-sponsored insurance plans. For example, under fee-for-service Medicare there is no limit on out-of-pocket expenditures and there are significant co-payments for some services. Consequently, many beneficiaries pay additional premiums for insurance to supplement Medicare (e.g., Medigap). How will the level of beneficiary out-of-pocket expenses be affected by efforts to control

Medicare spending? What is the impact of high out-of-pocket costs and gaps in Medicare coverage on beneficiaries' health and access to care? Medicare has been tasked by ACA with developing, expanding, or implementing a range of programs, demonstrations, and pilot programs related to accountable care organizations (ACO), bundled payments for care provided to a patient across various settings, reduced payments because of hospital readmissions and hospital acquired conditions, payments for care coordination, and value-based purchasing which can lead to lower medical costs and/or improved quality of care. How can these programs be designed to ensure that a sufficient number of providers will participate? How long will it take before results from these initiatives can be assessed? What elements are key to successful implementation (for example, adequate number of participating primary care providers, advanced and integrated information systems, changes to antitrust and antifraud legislation, and adequate financial incentives)? Can these models be successfully implemented for Medicare and also positively impact the private market for health care?

- In establishing the Center for Medicare and Medicaid Innovation as well as the Federal Coordinated Health Care Office under ACA, Congress provided options that can be used to experiment with new service delivery and payment options for beneficiaries of both Medicare and Medicaid. Will these changes help to maintain and improve quality of care while decreasing medical care costs to both the Medicaid and Medicare programs for dual eligible beneficiaries? What new approaches or authority might be necessary to ensure that acute and long-term care services are integrated, while maintaining or improving quality of care for dual eligible beneficiaries?
- Program integrity provisions in ACA increased resources, added new requirements, enhanced activities to prevent fraud and abuse, and increased uniformity in program integrity activities among Medicare, Medicaid, and CHIP. The Small Business and Jobs Act of 2010 (SBJA) provided additional appropriations to CMS for the development of predictive analytics technologies that could help to prevent fraudulent claims from being paid. Will these changes be sufficient to deter potentially fraudulent providers from entering the program, while at the same time not being so burdensome as to discourage legitimate providers from participating in Medicare? Will CMS, its contractors, and oversight agencies be better able to prevent

improper payments in the first place and reduce the reliance on the "pay-and-chase" approach? How much savings will be realized from these new authorities and activities; and how can this savings best be measured? Will additional authorities or new approaches be needed? Are program integrity resources appropriately allocated to all program areas, including Medicare Part C and D?

End Notes

[1] Also known as "customary, prevailing and reasonable charges," this method based physician payments on charges commonly used by physicians in a local community. The payment for a service was the lowest of (1) the physician's billed charge for the service, (2) the physician's customary charge for the service, or (3) the prevailing charge for that service in the community.

[2] ESRD is a stage of kidney impairment that appears to be irreversible and permanent, requiring a regular course of dialysis treatments or a kidney transplantation to maintain life.

[3] For more information, see CRS Report RL31966, *Overview of the Medicare Prescription Drug, Improvement, and Modernization Act of 2003.*

[4] For more information, see CRS Report RL34360, *P.L. 110-173: Provisions in the Medicare, Medicaid, and SCHIP Extension Act of 2007.*

[5] For more information, see CRS Report RL34592, *P.L. 110-275: The Medicare Improvements for Patients and Providers Act of 2008.*

[6] For more information, see CRS Report R41196, *Medicare Provisions in the Patient Protection and Affordable Care Act (PPACA): Summary and Timeline.*

[7] Groups of providers and suppliers who work together to manage and coordinate care for Medicare fee-for-service beneficiaries. See CRS Report R41474, *Accountable Care Organizations and the Medicare Shared Savings Program.*

[8] For a comprehensive discussion of the BCA, see CRS Report R41965, *The Budget Control Act of 2011*, by Bill Heniff Jr., Elizabeth Rybicki, and Shannon M. Mahan.

[9] Section 256(d) of the Balanced Budget and Emergency Deficit Control Act of 1985 (BBEDCA, P.L. 99-177) contains special rules for the Medicare program in case of a sequestration. While BBEDCA ordinarily limits reduction of certain Medicare spending to 4% under a sequestration order, the BCA limits the size of this reduction to 2%. See CRS Report R42050, *Budget "Sequestration" and Selected Program Exemptions and Special Rules*, coordinated by Karen Spar for additional detail.

[10] OMB will determine which parts of the Medicare program fall under the 2% cap and which could be subject to higher caps.

[11] Congressional Budget Office, *Estimated Impact of Automatic Budget Enforcement Procedures Specified in the Budget Control Act*, September 12, 2011, http://www.cbo.gov/ftp docs/124xx/doc12414/09-12-BudgetControlAct.pdf .

[12] For more information, see CRS Report RS22195, *Social Security Disability Insurance (SSDI) and Medicare: The 24- Month Waiting Period for SSDI Beneficiaries Under Age 65.*

[13] In 2012, all Part B enrollees, except for those subject to high income or late enrollment adjustments, pay the same premium amount of $99.90 per month. In 2011, because there was no Social Security cost-of-living adjustment (COLA) due to the economic slowdown, a

statutory hold-harmless provision prohibited established Medicare beneficiaries from Part B premium increases. The hold harmless protects an individual's Social Security benefit from a decrease as a result of a Part B premium increase. However, the provision did not apply to certain categories of beneficiaries, and some beneficiaries paid higher Part B premiums in 2011. See CRS Report R40561, *Interactions Between the Social Security COLA and Medicare Part B Premiums.*

[14] Starting in 2011, MA enrollees are only permitted to drop out of their MA plans and return to original Medicare during the first 45-day period of each calendar year. Though they are no longer allowed to switch to another MA plan as they were able to do previously, MA enrollees who use the 45-day period to disenroll from their MA plan may enroll in a stand-alone Part D prescription drug plan (PDP), or may elect to enroll in other non-Medicare Advantage private plan options, such as a Medicare Cost plan or a demonstration plan. MA enrollees will still be able to switch plans during special enrollment periods, such as when an MA enrollee moves outside his or her plan's service area or if an enrollee's MA plan is terminated.

[15] In addition to the yearly Medicare & You Handbook, http://www.medicare.gov/publications/pubs/pdf/10050.pdf, which is mailed to beneficiaries' homes, beneficiaries can consult http://www.Medicare.gov to find information such as the items and services covered under Medicare, cost sharing requirements, finding a participating medical provider or private health plan, and nursing home quality scores.

[16] If a Medicare beneficiary enrolls in a Private Fee-for-Service (PFFS) plan that does not provide drug coverage, he or she may enroll in a stand-alone Prescription Drug Plan (PDP). However, enrollees in other types of MA plans who want Part D prescription drug coverage must choose a Medicare Advantage Prescription Drug (MA-PD) plan, which is an MA plan that provides all Medicare required parts A, B, and D benefits. If a Medicare beneficiary enrolls in a local HMO or regional PPO that does not offer drug coverage, he or she does not have the option to enroll in a stand-alone PDP plan.

[17] Hospitals in the state of Maryland are exempt from the IPPS and are paid under a state-specific payment system.

[18] For additional information on skilled nursing facility benefits, see CRS Report R42401, *Medicare's Skilled Nursing Facility Primer: Benefit Basics and Issues*, by Scott R. Talaga.

[19] By October 1, 2013, the Secretary will be required to implement budget neutral revisions to the methodology for determining hospice payments for routine home care and other services. These revisions could include adjustments to the per diem payments reflecting differences in resources used during the course of an entire episode of hospice care.

[20] For details, see the Annual Reports of the Board of Trustees of the Federal Hospital Insurance and Federal Supplementary Medical Insurance Trust Funds, http://www.cms.hhs.gov/reportstrustfunds/.

[21] Certain durable medical equipment suppliers in competitive bidding areas are required to accept assignment.

[22] This "mental health parity" was introduced in MIPPA (P.L. 110-275). Beneficiaries are responsible for a 40% copayment for outpatient mental health services in 2012.

[23] For details, see CRS Report R40907, *Medicare Physician Payment Updates and the Sustainable Growth Rate (SGR) System*, by Jim Hahn and Janemarie Mulvey.

[24] The Temporary Payroll Tax Cut Continuation Act of 2011 (P.L. 112-78) included an override of the statutory SGR update for January and February 2012, and the Middle Class Tax Relief and Job Creation Act of 2012 (P.L. 112-96) maintained the payment freeze through the end of 2012.

[25] For details, see CRS Report R41196, *Medicare Provisions in the Patient Protection and Affordable Care Act (PPACA): Summary and Timeline*, coordinated by Patricia A. Davis.

[26] Social Security Act section 1862(a)(1)(A); 42 U.S.C. 1395y(a)(1)(A).

[27] U.S. Preventive Services Task Force, http://www.uspreventiveservicestaskforce.org/.

[28] A complete list of covered services, intervals, and limitations is available at CMS, overview of Medicare prevention, http://www.cms.gov/PrevntionGenInfo/.

[29] See General Accounting Office (GAO) report, "Medicare Payments for Oxygen," May 15, 1997, GAO-97-120R; HHS Office of the Inspector General report, "Medicare Home Oxygen Equipment: Cost and Servicing," September 2006, OEI-09-04-00420.

[30] For more information, see CRS Report R41211, *Medicare Durable Medical Equipment: The Competitive Bidding Program*, by Paulette C. Morgan.

[31] Biologics are generally derived from living organisms rather than inorganic chemical compounds.

[32] Additionally, starting in 2006, rural sole community hospitals (SCHs) receive an additional 7.1% in Medicare payments. Special payment protections apply to cancer hospitals, children's hospitals, small rural hospitals (that are not SCHs) with 100 or fewer beds, and SCHs.

[33] New, office-based procedures are services that are performed in physician offices at least 50% of the time. Payment is set at the lower of the ASC rate or the practice expense portion of the physician fee schedule payment rate.

[34] The Part D program was created by the Medicare Prescription Drug, Improvement, and Modernization Act of 2003 (P.L. 108-173), and began in 2006.

[35] The actual level of total covered Part D spending before reaching the catastrophic threshold will depend on whether the individual qualifies for the low-income subsidy and the portion of brand name and generic drugs purchased during the coverage gap.

[36] For additional information, see CRS Report R41196, *Medicare Provisions in the Patient Protection and Affordable Care Act (PPACA): Summary and Timeline*, coordinated by Patricia A. Davis.

[37] The ACA changed how these subsidies are treated for tax purposes. Employers currently can exclude the retiree drug subsidies from their gross income, as well as claim a business deduction for retiree prescription drug expenses. Beginning in 2013, the allowed deduction for retiree prescription drug coverage will be reduced by the amount of the federal drug subsidy received. For additional information, see CRS Report R41128, *Health-Related Revenue Provisions in the Patient Protection and Affordable Care Act (ACA)*, by Janemarie Mulvey.

[38] For more information, see http://www.cms.gov/MedicareContractingReform/ 02_Spotlight.asp#TopOfPage.

[39] For more information on Medicare contractors and Medicare fraud and abuse, see CRS Report RL34217, *Medicare Program Integrity: Activities to Protect Medicare from Payment Errors, Fraud, and Abuse*, by Cliff Binder.

[40] The Centers for Medicare & Medicaid Services, FY2011 Fee-for-Service Recovery Audit Program, November 23, 2011, https://www.cms.gov/Recovery-Audit-Program/02_Recent_Updates.asp#TopOfPage .

[41] Section 4241, "Use of Predictive Modeling and other Analytic Technologies to Identify and Prevent Waste, Fraud, and Abuse in the Medicare Fee-for-Service Program," of the Small Business and Jobs Act of 2010 (P.L. 111-240) authorized a one-time $100 million appropriation from the Medicare Trust Funds. The predictive modeling funding is available until expended. If certain interim objectives are not met by the predictive modeling

program, the Secretary may impose moratoriums on further expansion, until refinements or improvements are made.

[42] For more information, see http://innovations.cms.gov/.

[43] For more information on Medicare financing, see CRS Report R41436, *Medicare Financing*, by Patricia A. Davis.

[44] For more information, see CRS Report R41511, *The Independent Payment Advisory Board*, by Jim Hahn and Christopher M. Davis.

[45] 2012 Annual Report of the Boards of Trustees of the Federal Hospital Insurance and Federal Supplementary Medical Insurance Trust Funds, Table III.B4, p. 60, http://www.cms.hhs.gov/reportstrustfunds/. Note, the Medicare trustees generally report expenditures on a calendar year basis, while CBO reports on a fiscal year basis.

[46] For additional information on HI solvency estimates, see CRS Report RS20946, *Medicare: History of Insolvency Projections*, by Patricia A. Davis.

[47] 2012 Annual Report of the Boards of Trustees of the Federal Hospital Insurance and Federal Supplementary Medical Insurance Trust Funds, Table III.C4, p. 98, http://www.cms.hhs.gov/reportstrustfunds/.

[48] In 2010 and 2011, most Part B enrollees paid a monthly premium of $96.40. However, in 2010, new enrollees paid $110.50 per month and paid the same amount in 2011 due to the hold harmless provision. In 2011, new enrollees paid $115.40 per month. Those who didn't have Part B premiums deducted from a Social Security check (such as Federal Civil Service retirees, and those who have their premiums paid by Medicaid on their behalf) also paid $115.40 per month. For more information, see CRS Report R40561, *Interactions Between the Social Security COLA and Medicare Part B Premiums*, by Jim Hahn and Alison M. Shelton.

[49] The higher monthly premium amounts for 2012 are based on 2010 income levels and are (1) $139.90—for single beneficiaries with income $85,001-$107,000 or for each member of a couple filing jointly with income $170,001- $214,000; (2) $199.80—for single beneficiaries with income $107,001-$160,000 or for each member of a couple filing jointly with income $214,001-$320,000; (3) $259.70—for single beneficiaries with incomes $160,001-$214,000 and each member of a couple filing jointly with income $320,001-$428,000; and (4) $319.70—for single beneficiaries with incomes greater than $214,000 and each member of a couple filing jointly income above $428,000. ACA freezes these income thresholds through 2019 at 2010 levels, so potentially, as beneficiary income increases, more people may qualify for the higher income premium.

[50] 2012 Annual Report of the Boards of Trustees of the Federal Hospital Insurance and Federal Supplementary Medical Insurance Trust Funds, Table III.D3, p. 122, http://www.cms.hhs.gov/reportstrustfunds/.

[51] There is no "hold harmless" provision under Part D similar to that under Part B. Part D premium increases are not affected by Social Security cost-of-living adjustments.

[52] Starting in 2011, all MA plans are required to include a maximum out-of-pocket (OOP) limit determined by CMS. Prior to 2011, only MA regional plans were required to include a catastrophic cap on OOP spending.

[53] See CRS Report RL33202, *Medicaid: A Primer*, by Elicia J. Herz for additional information.

[54] In addition to individuals eligible for full Medicaid benefits, other low-income Medicare beneficiaries are entitled to limited benefits under the Medicare Savings Program (MSP). MSP includes three benefit categories each with different benefit levels: (1) Qualified Medicare Beneficiaries (QMBs), (2) Specified Low-Income Beneficiaries (SLMB), and (3) Qualified Individuals (QIs). For QMBs, state Medicaid programs pay Medicare Part B

premiums and Medicare cost-sharing (deductibles and co-payments) when beneficiaries' incomes are under 100% of the federal poverty level (FPL). For SLMBs, state Medicaid programs pay Part B premiums when beneficiaries' incomes are between 100% and 120% of the FPL. For QIs, Medicaid pays premiums when beneficiaries' incomes are between 120% and 135% of poverty. To be eligible for MSP, Medicare beneficiaries must also meet Medicaid's other eligibility requirements (e.g., meet citizenship or legal residency requirements).

[55] For additional information, see CRS Report RL30526, *Medicare Payment Policies*, coordinated by Paulette C. Morgan.

[56] Congressional Budget Office, Letter to the Honorable Dave Camp, December 9, 2011, *Estimate on H.R. 3630, the Middle Class Tax Relief and Job Creation Act of 2011, as introduced on December 9, 2011*, Table 2, http://www.cbo.gov/ftpdocs/126xx/doc12609/hr3630.pdf. Note: while the proposed legislation would have extended most of the provisions from January 2012 through December 2012, the CBO score reflects fiscal year estimates (October through September); therefore the CBO estimate shows increased costs in both FY2012 and FY2013.

Index

F

G

H

I

J

K

L

M

N

O

P

Q

R

S

T

U

V

W